T0238955

Congenital Hip Disease in Adults

George Hartofilakidis • George C. Babis
Kalliopi Lampropoulou-Adamidou

Congenital Hip Disease in Adults

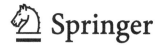 Springer

George Hartofilakidis, MD, FACS
Orthopaedic Department
Medical School
National and Kapodistrian University
Athens
Greece

George C. Babis, MD, DSc
2nd Orthopaedic Department
Medical School
National and Kapodistrian University
Nea Ionia General Hospital
"Konstantopoulion"
Athens
Greece

Kalliopi Lampropoulou-Adamidou, MD,
MSc
3rd Orthopaedic Department
National and Kapodistrian University
KAT General Hospital
Athens
Greece

ISBN 978-88-470-5877-4   ISBN 978-88-470-5492-9   (eBook)
DOI 10.1007/978-88-470-5492-9
Springer Milan Heidelberg New York Dordrecht London

Printed on acid-free paper

Springer is part of Springer Science+Business Media (www.springer.com)

Preface

This work is presented on the basis of knowledge and experience acquired in the long course of my surgical practice on the complex problem of congenital abnormalities of the hip. A lot of this experience has been reported in a series of lectures and international publications, and is summarised in this book.

Searching and extracting information from a voluminous record over a long past was an arduous task. In this regard, the contribution of the co-authors, George C. Babis and Kalliopi Lampropoulou-Adamidou, was most important. Having an extensive experience on the subject, Professor George C. Babis provided valuable advice and suggestions in reviewing the manuscript. Review of the current literature, writing of certain parts of the manuscript and preparation and organisation of the material by Kalliopi Lampropoulou-Adamidou were critical contributions. Editing of special sections of the work by Professor Spyros M. Vratsanos is gratefully acknowledged.

The basic anatomy and certain aspects of osteoarthritis (OA) of the hip are discussed in the two introductory chapters. The distinction of OA of the hip, as idiopathic and secondary, is helpful to the surgeon in estimating the development in each type and in suggesting the appropriate approach.

The main cause of the secondary OA of the hip is the congenital hip disease (CHD), representing about 40 % of all OA cases of the hip. Understanding the classification of CHD in dysplasia, low dislocation and high dislocation, and being informed of the natural history of each type is crucial for the management of the disease, for which, in recent years total hip replacement (THR) has been the main approach. Particularly significant is the appreciation of the value of indications for THR. Furthermore, preoperative assessment is important. Regarding surgical techniques, the authors' experience and internationally reported techniques are presented.

The importance of a systematic follow-up for a timely revision is emphasised. Such revision may be successful and prevents extensive bone destruction.

Two case studies are included, one demonstrates the approaches and techniques used in handling difficult cases; the other highlights the radical improvement of the quality of life of patients born with severe deformities of the hip joint, after THR.

A large number of figures copied from our archive and previous publications are included, as a necessary and efficient complement of the information provided by the text.

In leaving this work in the hands of my colleagues, I believe that its detailed information on a subject not efficiently covered in the literature may be helpful in their efforts to further advance the art of reconstructive surgery of the hip.

Athens, Greece   George Hartofilakidis

Contents

1 **The Hip: Basic Anatomy** 1
   References 2

2 **Osteoarthritis of the Hip** 3
   References 10

3 **Congenital Hip Disease: General Aspects, Terminology
   and Classification** 11
   3.1 General Aspects 11
   3.2 Terminology 12
   3.3 Classification................................... 15
   References 27

4 **Epidemiology, Demographics and Natural History** 29
   4.1 Epidemiology and Demographics.................... 29
   4.2 Natural History 30
   References 43

5 **Treatment Options, Except Total Hip Replacement:
   Conservative Management and Osteotomies** 45
   5.1 Conservative Management 45
   5.2 Osteotomies 45
   References 51

6 **Total Hip Replacement: Indications and Preoperative
   Assessment** 53
   6.1 Indications..................................... 53
   6.2 Preoperative Assessment 56
   References 61

7 **Technical Considerations** 63
   7.1 Wide Exposure 63
   7.2 Restoration of the Normal Centre of Rotation 64
   7.3 Reconstruction of the Acetabulum 65
   7.4 Classic Cotyloplasty Technique 67
   7.5 Reconstruction of the Femur 69
   References 74

8   Complications and Results   77
    8.1   Complications   77
    8.2   Results   78
        8.2.1   Authors' Related Publications   81
    References   84

9   Difficult Cases   87

10   Timing for Revision   113
    References   129

11   Quality of Life After Total Hip Replacement   131
    References   163

12   Conclusive Messages   165

Index   167

The joint of the hip develops from the cartilaginous anlage at 4–6 weeks of the embryonic development. At 7 weeks of gestation, a cleft develops between pre-cartilaginous cells defining the femoral head and acetabulum, and at 11 weeks, the hip joint formation is complete. Then, the femoral head is encircled by the acetabulum and it is difficult to dislocate [1].

The hip is the biggest and more stable joint in the human body. It is formed from the femoral head and a deep cavity, with raised bone margins, the acetabulum (Figs. 1.1, 1.2 and 1.3). It is a typical ball-and-socket joint. The depth of the acetabulum increased by the fibrocartilaginous labrum which is attached circumferentially to the bony rim providing 170° coverage of the femoral head. The bony rim of the acetabulum is interrupted at its lower part to form the acetabular notch, which is then bridged by the extension of the labrum, the transverse ligament. The acetabular branch of the obturator artery passes under the transverse ligament to enter the ligamentum teres. The inferior part of the acetabulum is referred to as acetabular fossa, being the thinnest part of the acetabular floor. The laminate-shaped articular cartilage of the acetabulum covers its periphery, while acetabular fossa remains without cartilage. The head of the femur, that forms two-thirds of a sphere, is covered by articular cartilage, except of the fossa for the attachment of ligamentum teres.

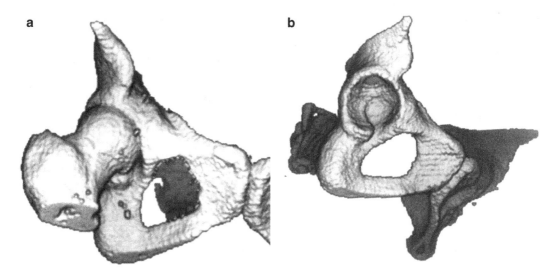

a

b

Fig. 1.1 3D-CT scans of a normal hip. (**a**) With and (**b**) without the femoral head

G. Hartofilakidis et al., *Congenital Hip Disease in Adults*,
DOI 10.1007/978-88-470-5492-9_1, © Springer-Verlag Italia 2014

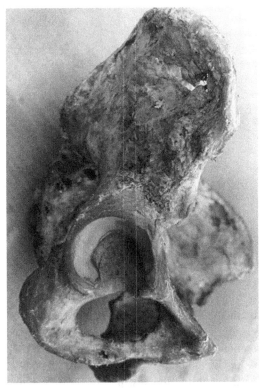

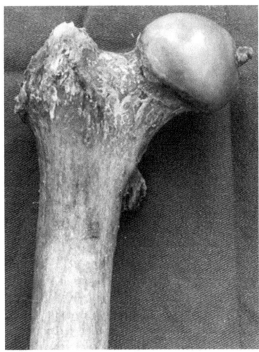

Fig. 1.3 The normal femur in a cadaveric specimen

Fig. 1.2 The normal acetabulum in a cadaveric specimen

In a normal hip, the acetabulum is positioned approximately 45° caudally and 15° anteriorly. The angle between the femoral shaft and the neck of the femur is approximately 135°, and the distance between the centre of the femoral head and the line passing through the long axis of the femur represents the offset of the hip joint.

The teardrop is a very important radiographic sign at the most distal part of the acetabulum. The lateral lip corresponds to the floor of the acetabular fossa and the medial lip to the internal wall of the acetabulum.

Clinically, the hip is the joint with the greater range of motion. It has flexion 120–130°, extension 10–20°, abduction 20–30°, adduction 30–40°, external rotation 30–40° and internal rotation 20–30° [2–4].

References

1. Wheeless CR (2011) Embryology of the hip. Wheeless' textbook of orthopaedics. http://www.wheelessonline.com/ortho/12586. Last updated 9 January 2013
2. Wasielewski RC (2007) The hip. In: Callaghan JJ, Rosenberg AG, Rubash HE (eds) The adult hip, vol 1, 2nd edn. Lippincott Williams and Wilkins, Philadelphia, pp 51–52
3. Resnick D, Niwayama S (1998) Hip. Osseous anatomy. In: Resnick D, Niwayama S (eds) Diagnosis of bone and joint disorders. WB Saunders, London, pp 100–101
4. Eftekhar N (1993) Applied surgical anatomy. In: Eftekhar N (ed) Total hip arthroplasty, vol 1. Mosby, St. Louis, pp 17–50

Osteoarthritis (OA), a common degenerative disease of the hip joint, is a matter of great concern among orthopaedic surgeons. Most adult patients seen in everyday practice, with pain, limping or stiffness of the hip, are suffering from OA and less commonly from other pathological causes such as rheumatoid arthritis, avascular necrosis, trauma etc.

The reported incidence of the hip OA in the general population varies considerably, depending on the different methods used for the selection of the sample, the diagnostic criteria applied and the race and age of the patients participating in different studies [1–4].

Two types of hip OA are recognised: idiopathic, when the underlying cause cannot be determined, and secondary, when a predisposed cause is well defined. Although for many years a controversy existed for the subsistence of idiopathic OA [5–7], recent studies by Karachalios et al. [4] and Dagenais et al. [8] suggest that the idiopathic OA is rather common among adult population. The exact incidence of each type of OA is a subject of controversy [3, 4, 9–12], with idiopathic OA rarely found in Asians [4, 8, 9, 11], a race with high incidence of secondary OA due to congenital hip disease (CHD) [1, 13].

A systematic review of the English literature on the prevalence of radiographic idiopathic OA summarised that although the reported estimates varied considerably among different studies, radiographic idiopathic OA is present in approximately 5–10 % of the general adult population [8]. Yet, it is found that in multiracial countries there is a virtual absence of idiopathic OA in Asians and low rates in Black and Spanish populations [14].

We studied a series of 660 osteoarthritic hips in 465 patients and found that a considerable number of hips (272 hips, 41 %) had idiopathic OA, in the absence of any anatomical abnormality (see also Chap. 4) and we concluded that idiopathic OA does exist and is common [15].

The direction of migration of the femoral head and the evolution of the degenerative changes are used as criteria to classify idiopathic OA [12, 16–23]. Most of the authors agree that two main types of head migration can be clearly recognised: eccentric, when the femoral head migrates superolaterally, and concentric, when migration occurs medially. In our study, eccentric OA was four times more common than concentric, with the ratio between women and men being 4:1, slightly more in the eccentric type.

Idiopathic OA occurs in patients with previous anatomically normal hips usually at the age of 50–60 years. Eccentric OA has a bad prognosis and has a rapid deterioration requiring surgery within few years (Figs. 2.1 and 2.2). Concentric OA has a better prognosis and has a slower deterioration requiring surgery usually after 10 or more years (Figs. 2.3 and 2.4).

G. Hartofilakidis et al., *Congenital Hip Disease in Adults*,
DOI 10.1007/978-88-470-5492-9_2, © Springer-Verlag Italia 2014

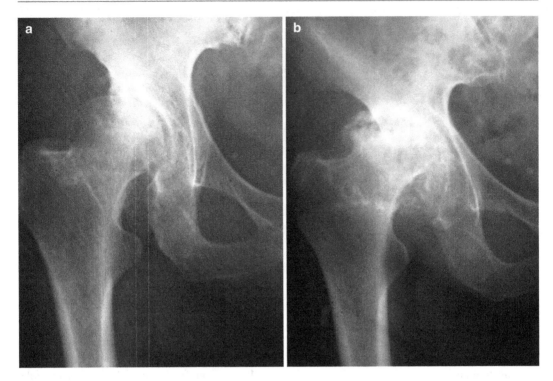

Fig. 2.1 The evolution of degenerative changes in a hip with eccentric idiopathic OA in a period of 4 years. (**a**) Radiograph taken when the patient was 56 years old. She had mild symptoms. (**b**) Rapid deterioration within 4 years. The patient had severe pain and limping

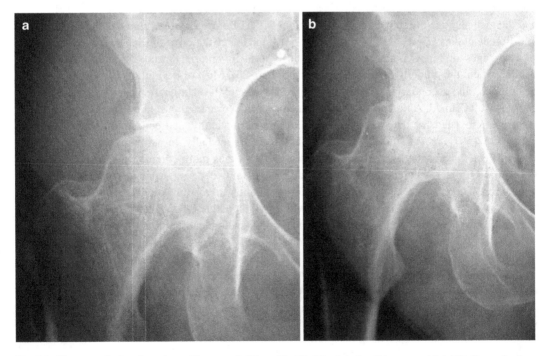

Fig. 2.2 The case of a female patient with eccentric idiopathic OA. The deterioration was rapid. (**a**) Radiograph when the patient was 62 years old. (**b**) Two years later, radiograph and patient's clinical picture worsen dramatically

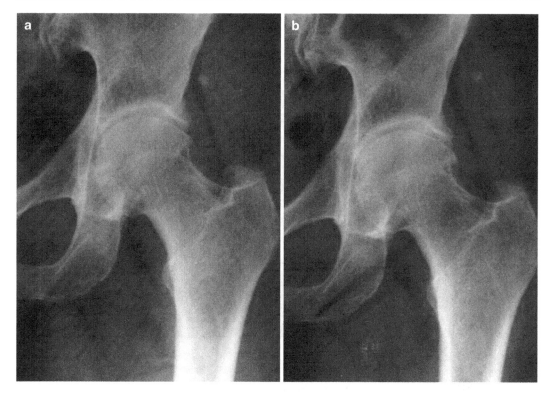

Fig. 2.3 Images illustrate the case of a male patient with concentric OA. (**a**) Radiograph when the patient was 56 years old and had minor symptoms. (**b**) At the age of 74, 16 years later, patient had slow clinical and radiographic deterioration

A patient with unilateral idiopathic OA has approximately 30 % possibility to develop idiopathic OA in the opposite hip several years later (Fig. 2.5) [24], a fact pointing to systemic biological factors that predispose both hips to develop OA.

The most common cause of secondary OA is CHD, which is the main topic of this book. Less common causes are osteochondritis and slipped capital epiphysis and for some authors femoroacetabular impingement (FAI).

It was as early as in 1936 when Smith-Petersen first proposed FAI as a cause of OA of the hip and described its surgical treatment (Fig. 2.6) [25]. However, only recently, orthopaedic surgeons were interested in the subject, following the work of Ganz et al. in 2003 [26]. Early surgical treatment has been recommended in order to avoid the development of OA [27]. The procedures advised included periacetabular osteotomy, dislocation of the hip or mini-

anterior approach and osteochondroplasty and arthroscopy for isolated labrum repair or in combination with osteochondroplasty. This concept gained wide acceptance and a substantial number of publications followed. Nevertheless, recently, doubts and concerns were raised even by Ganz et al. [28], the supporters of this theory, questioning whether all patients with morphological abnormalities, indicative of FAI, would necessarily develop OA, and suggesting long-term radiological studies of asymptomatic young adults to demonstrate both the negative and positive power of the hypothesis. In this connection, Brand, the former Editor of CORR, wrote "We do not know whether current procedures for FAI will delay the development of OA in the middle age and beyond" [29].

In an effort to answer these questions we examined the long-term (10–40 years) radiographic outcome of 96 asymptomatic hips in people with a mean age of 49 years (16–65) who

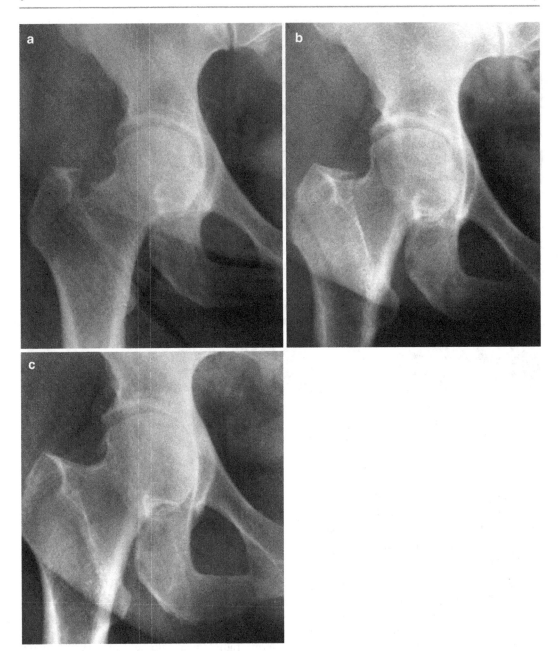

Fig. 2.4 Images illustrate the case of a female patient with concentric idiopathic OA. Slow deterioration is shown from the age of (**a**) 50 to (**b**) 60 and (**c**) 70. Patient is still tolerating symptoms

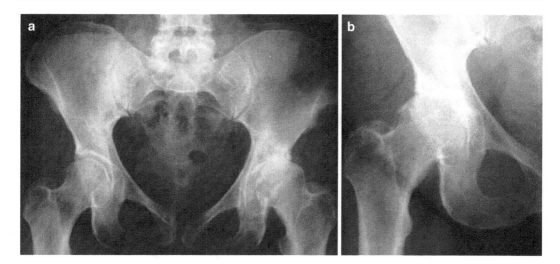

Fig. 2.5 Images illustrate the case of a female patient with unilateral idiopathic OA. (**a**) Radiograph when the patient was 51 years old. Left hip presents eccentric idiopathic OA. Right hip appears normal. (**b**) Twenty years later, when the patient was 71 years old, the right hip also developed eccentric idiopathic OA

had radiographic evidence of FAI [30]. The results of this study showed that 79 hips (82 %) remained OA-free for a mean of 19 years (10–40) (Figs. 2.7 and 2.8), and only 17 hips (18 %) developed OA after a mean time of 12 years.

We believe that in young patients, especially those with intense sport activities, who have pain in the hip and radiographic evidence of FAI, the symptoms probably originate from labrum tears or mere synovitis. If these symptoms do not subside with conservative measures, arthroscopy is the best treatment to repair the labrum damage. It would be of interest to establish whether reconstruction of the damaged labrum, associated with pistol-grip deformity, should be combined with osteochondroplasty, at the time of arthroscopy.

Congenital hip disease remains the main cause of secondary OA of the hip. In this volume, we are intending to inform the surgeons concerned with CHD about terminology and classification of the disease, its natural history and treatment with total hip replacement including indications, preoperative assessment and techniques adjusted to the different types of the disease.

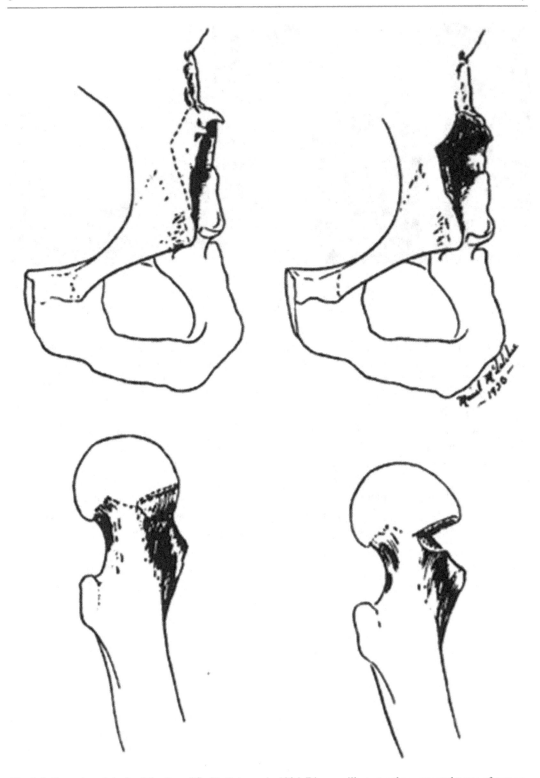

Fig. 2.6 From the original publication of Smith-Petersen in 1936. Diagram illustrates the suggested types of surgery, which are similar to those used nowadays

Fig. 2.7 Images illustrate the case of a male patient with asymptomatic pistol-grip deformity of both hips. (**a**) Radiograph taken at the age of 43 for unrelated to the hips pathology. (**b**) Forty-two years later, hips remained asymptomatic without evidence of OA

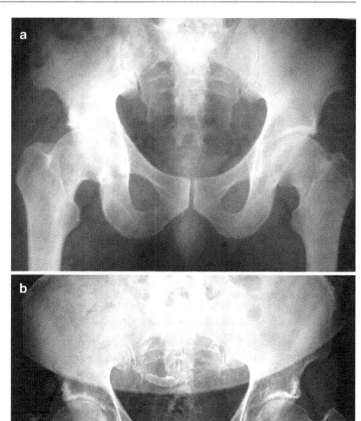

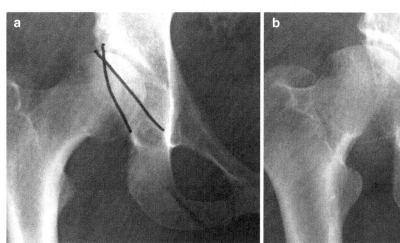
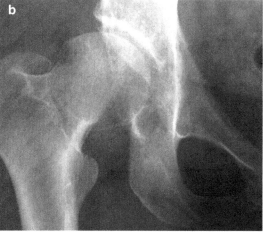

Fig. 2.8 Images illustrate the case of a female patient with asymptomatic right hip. (**a**) Radiograph taken at the age of 33. Note that the hip is in varus (120° NS angle) and the acetabulum in retroversion. (**b**) Twenty-four years later, the hip remained OA-free

References

1. Aronson J (1986) Osteoarthritis of the young adult hip: etiology and treatment. Instr Course Lect 35: 119–128
2. Hoaglund FT, Yau AC, Wong WL (1973) Osteoarthritis of the hip and other joints in southern Chinese in Hong Kong. J Bone Joint Surg Am 55(3):545–557
3. Jorring K (1980) Osteoarthritis of the hip. Epidemiology and clinical role. Acta Orthop Scand 51(3): 523–530
4. Karachalios T, Karantanas AH, Malizos K (2007) Hip osteoarthritis: what the radiologist wants to know. Eur J Radiol 63(1):36–48
5. Murray RO (1965) The aetiology of primary osteoarthritis of the hip. Br J Radiol 38(455):810–824
6. Stulberg SD, Cordell LD, Harris WH, Ramsey PL, MacEwen GD (1975) Unrecognized childhood hip disease: a major cause of idiopathic osteoarthritis of the hip. In: The hip: proceedings of the third open scientific meeting of the Hip Society. CV Mosby, St Louis, pp 212–228
7. Harris WH (1986) Etiology of osteoarthritis of the hip. Clin Orthop Relat Res 213:20–33
8. Dagenais S, Garbedian S, Wai EK (2009) Systematic review of the prevalence of radiographic primary hip osteoarthritis. Clin Orthop Relat Res 467(3):623–637
9. Hoaglund FT, Shiba R, Newberg AH, Leung KY (1985) Diseases of the hip. A comparative study of Japanese Oriental and American white patients. J Bone Joint Surg Am 67(9):1376–1383
10. Dutowsky JP (1998) Miscellaneous nontraumatic disorders. In: Canale ST (ed) Campbell's operative orthopaedics, 9th edn. Mosby, St Louis, p 818
11. Nakamura S, Ninomiya S, Nakamura T (1989) Primary osteoarthritis of the hip joint in Japan. Clin Orthop Relat Res 241:190–196
12. Resnick D, Niwayama G (1988) Degenerative joint disease in specific locations. In: Diagnosis of bone and joint disorders. WB Saunders, Philadelphia, pp 1426–1442
13. Hartofilakidis G (1997) Survival of the Charnley low-friction arthroplasty. A 12-24-year follow-up of 276 cases. Acta Orthop Scand Suppl 275:27–29
14. Hoaglund FT, Oishi CS, Gialamas GG (1995) Extreme variations in racial rates of total hip arthroplasty for primary coxarthrosis: a population-based study in San Francisco. Ann Rheum Dis 54(2): 107–110
15. Hartofilakidis G, Karachalios T (2003) Idiopathic osteoarthritis of the hip: incidence, classification, and natural history of 272 cases. Orthopedics 26(2):161–166
16. Altman RD (1987) Criteria for the classification of osteoarthritis of the knee and hip. Scand J Rheumatol Suppl 65:31–39
17. Bissacotti JF, Ritter MA, Faris PM, Keating EM, Cates HE (1994) A new radiographic evaluation of primary osteoarthritis. Orthopedics 17(10):927–930
18. Cameron HU, Macnab I (1975) Observations on osteoarthritis of the hip joint. Clin Orthop Relat Res 108:31–40
19. Gofton JP (1971) Studies in osteoarthritis of the hip. I. Classification. Can Med Assoc J 104(8):679–683
20. Gofton JP (1983) A classification of osteoarthritis of the hip and its relevance to pathogenesis. J Rheumatol S9:65–66
21. Hermodsson I (1970) Roentgen appearance of coxarthrosis. Relation between the anatomy, pathologic changes, and roentgen appearance. Acta Orthop Scand 41(2):169–187
22. Macys JR, Bullough PG, Wilson PD Jr (1980) Coxarthrosis: a study of the natural history based on a correlation of clinical, radiographic, and pathologic findings. Semin Arthritis Rheum 10(1):66–80
23. Wroblewski BM, Charnley J (1982) Radiographic morphology of the osteoarthritic hip. J Bone Joint Surg Br 64(5):568–569
24. Vossinakis IC, Georgiades G, Kafidas D, Hartofilakidis G (2008) Unilateral hip osteoarthritis: can we predict the outcome of the other hip? Skeletal Radiol 37(10):911–916
25. Smith-Petersen MN, Boston MD (1936) Treatment of malum coxae senilis, old slipped upper femoral epiphysis, intrapelvic protrusion of the acetabulum, and coxa Plana by means of acetabuloplasty. J Bone Joint Surg Am 18:869–880
26. Ganz R, Parvizi J, Beck M, Leunig M, Notzli H, Siebenrock KA (2003) Femoroacetabular impingement: a cause for osteoarthritis of the hip. Clin Orthop Relat Res 417:112–120
27. Parvizi J, Leunig M, Ganz R (2007) Femoroacetabular impingement. J Am Acad Orthop Surg 15(9):561–570
28. Ganz R, Leunig M, Leunig-Ganz K, Harris WH (2008) The etiology of osteoarthritis of the hip: an integrated mechanical concept. Clin Orthop Relat Res 466(2):264–272
29. Brand RA (2009) Femoroacetabular impingement: current status of diagnosis and treatment: Marius Nygaard Smith-Petersen, 1886-1953. Clin Orthop Relat Res 467(3):605–607
30. Hartofilakidis G, Bardakos NV, Babis GC, Georgiades G (2011) An examination of the association between different morphotypes of femoroacetabular impingement in asymptomatic subjects and the development of osteoarthritis of the hip. J Bone Joint Surg Br 93(5):580–586

Congenital Hip Disease: General Aspects, Terminology and Classification

3

3.1 General Aspects

The use of ultrasound as a screening test in the newborn has allowed earlier diagnosis and treatment, with a better prognosis, for congenital hip disease (CHD) [1]. However, orthopaedic surgeons who specialise in adult reconstruction surgery often face the problem of osteoarthritis (OA) secondary to CHD in adult patients. These cases could be of different severity and are usually the result of late diagnosis and treatment in areas where early screening and treatment were not effective or in patients in whom treatment had failed in childhood [2].

Congenital disease is the main cause of secondary OA of the hip (Fig. 3.1). Other causes such as osteochondritis (Fig. 3.2) and slipped capital femoral epiphysis (SCFE) (Fig. 3.3) are much less common. Femoroacetabular impingement (FAI) has also been considered as a cause of early OA (Fig. 2.7). However, there is no clinical confirmation to support this hypothesis [3, 4].

Hip pain and limping are the cardinal symptoms leading young adults with secondary OA due to CHD to the specialised surgeons. Often, patients' complaints include early fatigue and pain in the back and/or the knees.

Before the introduction of total hip replacement (THR), patients with CHD were doomed to disability during all their lives. Femoral and pelvic osteotomies had limited indications and short-term satisfactory results (Figs. 3.4 and 3.5). The introduction of THR, the revolutionary operation of the past century, radically

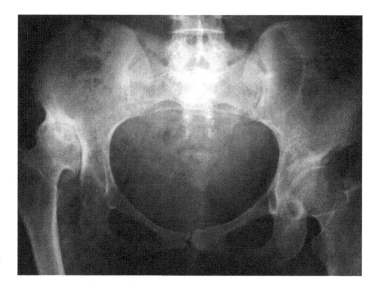

Fig. 3.1 A 30-year-old female with bilateral secondary OA due to CHD

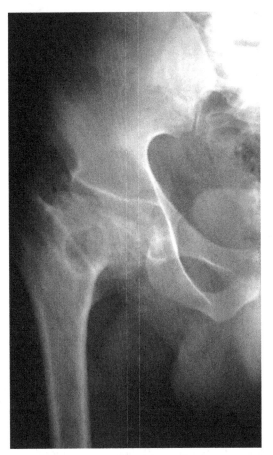

Fig. 3.2 A 32-year-old male with secondary OA of the right hip due to osteochondritis

improved the quality of life of these patients, especially of young females with severe types of CHD, presenting a special group of patients with problematic life since birth. Apart from their young age, these patients have several psychological disorders, as anxiety and depression, since their early childhood. Having been born and raised with this deformity in an able-bodied privileged society have had their lives affected in a fundamental way. In addition to experiences of multiple and prolonged treatments in early childhood, these patients describe traumatic experiences, especially during their developmental years, impacting them socially, mentally and emotionally. Treatment with THR makes the change in quality of their life much more dramatic. It is of particular interest, how some patients describe certain life experiences after surgery: "I felt that I was born again", "I see

myself in the mirror and I don't believe my eyes", "Men started paying attention to me", "Some people talk about a miracle", "I work, travel, I have fun without a concern about my hips problem", "I developed faith in myself" (see more details in Chap. 11). Even patients who underwent several revisions had enjoyed life free of pain with function improvement for a reasonable period of time [5].

Orthopaedic surgeons who treat adult patients with CHD should be familiar with its terminology and be able to recognise the anatomical abnormalities. Most importantly to know the absolute indications for THR, carry out through preoperative planning, reconstruct the hip using the appropriate surgical technique and implants and finally be able to anticipate the clinical outcome and avoid complications.

This volume aims to provide the surgeons concerned with CHD with relevant information based mainly on the authors' experience.

3.2   Terminology

For better communication, treatment planning and evaluation of results of different treatments, there is a need for an agreed terminology, which covers the entire spectrum of congenital deformities of the hip.

The congenital nature of the disease has been recognised, even before availability of radiographs, when Dupuytren [6], in 1826, observed some newborn infants with displacement of the head of the femur from the acetabulum. He named this condition "congenital displacement". Dupuytren's recognition of the congenital nature of the deformity has been accepted as original. In 1897, Phelps [7], based on anatomical specimens, also considered that the majority of such cases are really dislocations at birth. Since that time, in many other pioneer works with anatomical dissections and studies of the pathologic features at open operations, the authors had accepted the congenital nature of the deformity [8–13].

The term "congenital displacement" proposed by Dupuytren was slightly modified to "congenital dislocation of the hip", a term that dominated

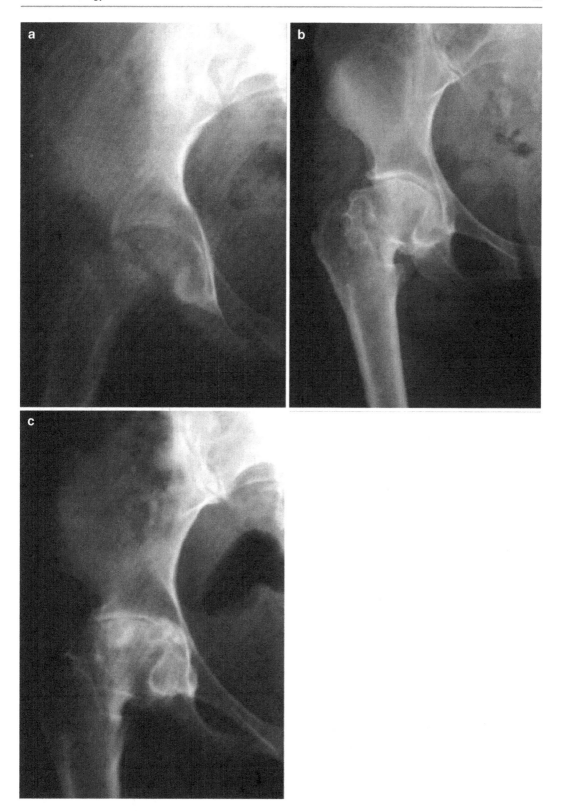

Fig. 3.3 Female patient with a chronic slipped capital epiphysis treated with a subtrochanteric osteotomy at the age of 12. (**a**) Preoperative radiograph. (**b**) Radiograph taken when the patient was 31 years old. She was slightly limping without pain. (**c**) At the age of 37, patient had developed secondary OA. She had severe pain and was heavily limping

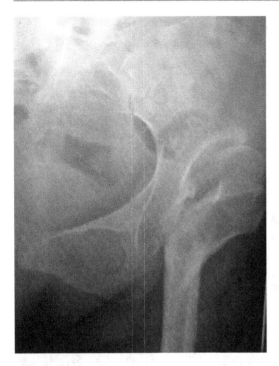

Fig. 3.4 This patient at the age of 17, in 1962, had a Schanz subtrochanteric osteotomy, which caused great technical difficulties when patient came for hip replacement, 15 years later

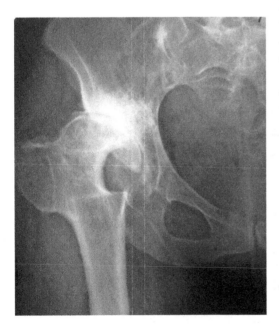

Fig. 3.5 A 42-year-old female with advanced secondary OA of the hip due to CHD. At the age of 31, in 1970, she had a McMurray subtrochanteric osteotomy with no clear indications

among orthopaedics, paediatricians and other physicians for decades. However, it was later recognised that the use of this term led to considerable confusion in understanding the underlying deformities and in communication between physicians, and its accuracy became questionable. The congenital nature of the deformity has not been disputed by the majority of authors, but it was recognised that variable pathologies that existed at birth and progressed in adult life were not necessarily dislocations. During the following years the literature on the pathogenesis and terminology of congenital dislocation of the hip were replete with contradictions and uncertainties. In 1989, in his brief report, Klisic emphasised that congenital dislocation is a misleading term, when used for the total spectrum of the deformity [14]. Instead, he recommended the use of the term "developmental displacement". Though many authors and the American Academy of Orthopaedic Surgeons accepted the change in wording of congenital to developmental, on the other hand, they replaced the wording of displacement, proposed by Klisic, with that of dysplasia, and a new term "developmental dysplasia of the hip" was established. Nonetheless, despite the latest effort for an appropriate definition covering the total spectrum of the disease, inaccuracies still persist, reflecting mainly the confusion as to the original cause. Specifically, the term developmental is not descriptive of the congenital nature of the deformity, while an indiscriminate use of the term dysplasia does not reflect the variety of underlying pathology. Thus, unfortunately, from a deficient term "congenital dislocation", we ended up with a non-specific and unsuitable one "developmental dysplasia of the hip", without convincing arguments for the change. Developmental has the meaning of evolving, gradually changing and progressing. However, in this case, the disorder is congenital in origin – the primary abnormality originates in utero and developmental in nature, which is a dynamic process. On the other hand, the term "dysplasia", a mixed Greek word, composed by the word "bad" and "form", can be reserved for the mildest types of hip deformities, in contrast to the most severe types of hip dislocations,

Fig. 3.6 By using the term "dysplasia", for both these hips, inaccuracy of description is obvious. Note that the right femoral head articulates with a false acetabulum, and the left with the true acetabulum

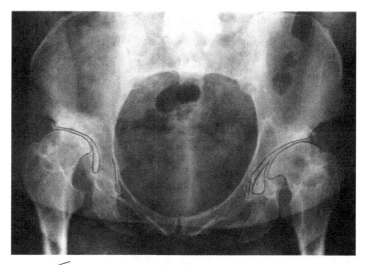

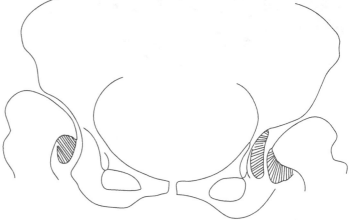

avoiding confusion and diagnostic inaccuracies [15] (Fig. 3.6). Furthermore, the term "subluxation", used for the description of infant hips, should not be used in adults, because this simply refers to the degree of the displacement of the femoral head, without defining anatomical abnormalities at the site (Fig. 3.7).

Authors' suggestion is to use the term "congenital hip disease" for the entire spectrum of the deformities (Fig. 3.8).

3.3 Classification

An internationally accepted classification system improves communication, planning of treatment and comparison of results of different treatments, by avoiding inclusion of dissimilar cases within the same series. For a classification system to be useful in clinical practice, it should be accurate, precisely describing the underlying pathological anatomy, simple and easy to memorise. Several classification systems have been used to describe the different types of congenital hip disease (CHD) in adults. The most commonly used are those of Crowe et al. [16] and Hartofilakidis et al. [17, 18]. Other classification systems are those by Eftekhar [19] and Kerboull [20] (Table 3.1).

Crowe et al. classification is based on three anatomical landmarks, identified in a whole pelvis radiograph (Fig. 3.9): (1) the height of the pelvis, (2) the medial head-neck junction and (3) the lower part of the teardrop.

The vertical distance between the reference interteardrop line and the head-neck junction

Fig. 3.7 Right and left hip show almost the same degree of subluxation of the femoral head. However, the underlying anatomical abnormalities differ

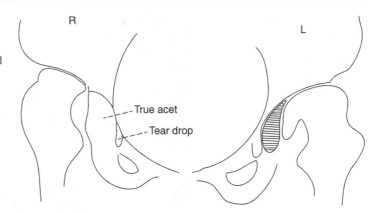

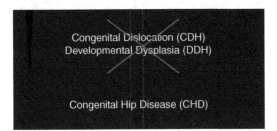

Fig. 3.8 Congenital hip disease is the term suggested by the authors

indicates the degree of subluxation (proximal migration of the femoral head), and the one between the line connecting the ischial tuberosities and the iliac crests indicates the height of the pelvis. Four types of dislocation are described according to the a/b value: type I, when proximal migration of the femoral head is less than 10 % of pelvic height ($a/b<0.1$); type II, when it is 10–15 % $0.1<a/b<0.15$; type III, 15–20 % $0.15<a/b<0.2$; and type IV, when it is more than 20 % ($a/b>0.2$).

Hartofilakidis et al. classification, based on radiographic and intraoperative criteria, recognises three main types of increasing severity (Figs. 3.10, 3.11, 3.12 and 3.13): dysplasia (type A), in which the femoral head articulates with the true acetabulum, despite the degree of subluxation; low dislocation (type B), in which the femoral head articulates with a false acetabulum that partially covers the true acetabulum to a varying degree; and high dislocation (type C), where the femoral head has migrated superiorly and posteriorly in relation to the true acetabulum and may articulate with a hollow in the iliac wing, which resembles a false acetabulum, or move freely within the gluteal muscles [17, 18].

In dysplastic hips, the acetabulum presents a deficiency of the superior segment and a secondary shallowing due to the formation of a large osteophyte that covers the acetabular fossa. In low dislocation, the inferior part of the false acetabulum is an osteophyte that resembles the superior rim of the true acetabulum. The visible part of the true acetabulum has a narrow opening, anterior and posterior segmental deficiency and inadequate depth. In the majority of cases, there is also increased anteversion. In high dislocation, the true acetabulum is hypoplastic and triangular in shape. It has a segmental deficiency of its entire rim, a narrow opening, inadequate depth and excessive anteversion (Figs. 3.14 and 3.15).

The femoral head in the dysplastic hip, is initially spherical but, as the deformity progresses, becomes elliptical and elongated, due to the formation of marginal osteophytes. The femoral neck and the diaphysis are within the range of normal anatomy. In low dislocation, the femoral head is often large and elliptical in shape also due to the formation of marginal osteophytes. The femoral neck is short, occasionally is anteverted, and the diaphysis is narrow. In high dislocation, the femoral head is small, especially when it does not articulate with a false acetabulum. The femoral neck is short always with increased anteversion and the lesser trochanter lies more anteriorly than normal. The diaphysis is hypoplastic with an extreme narrowing of the canal and with a thin cortex (Fig. 3.16).

Table 3.1 Details of classification systems for congenital hip disease

Author(s)	Hartofilakidis et al.	Crowe et al.	Eftekhar	Kerboull
Types of increasing severity	Dysplasia	I, <50 %	Dysplasia	Anterior
		II, 50–75 %		
	Low dislocation B1	III, 75–100 %	Intermediate dislocation	Intermediate
	Low dislocation B2			
	High dislocation C1	IV, >100 %	High dislocation	Posterior
	High dislocation C2		Old unreduced dislocation	
Characteristic features	Description of anatomical abnormalities	Proximal migration/ height of femoral head	Degree of subluxation	Direction of subluxation

Fig. 3.9 The Crowe classification relies on the percentage of the height of the dislocation (a) in relation to the height of the pelvis (b)

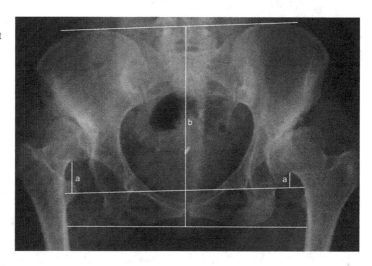

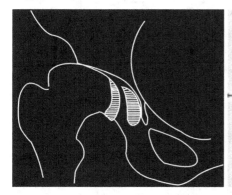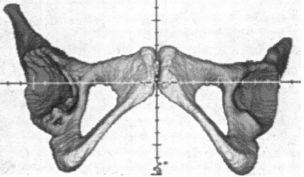

Fig. 3.10 Type A (dysplasia) of Hartofilakidis classification. The femoral head is contained within the original acetabulum. Note the large osteophyte that covers the acetabular fossa and the medial marginal osteophyte of the femoral head (capital drop)

Previous osteotomies may result in residual angular deformities of the proximal femur which can make the reconstruction more challenging (Fig. 3.17) [21].

The Hartofilakidis et al. classification corresponds to the Crowe et al. classification as follows: dysplastic hips correspond to Crowe's type I and II hips, low dislocation corresponds to

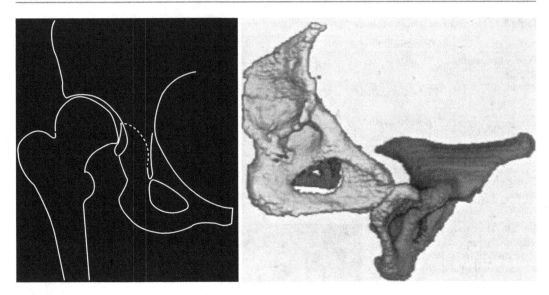

Fig. 3.11 Type B (low dislocation). The femoral head articulates with a false acetabulum that partially covers the true acetabulum

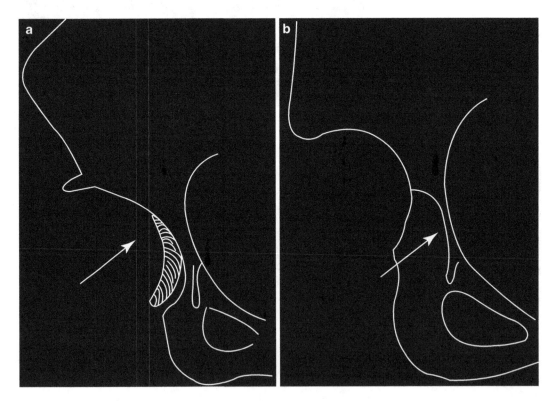

Fig. 3.12 Diagrams illustrate the position of true acetabulum (*arrows*) (**a**) in dysplastic and (**b**) low dislocated hips

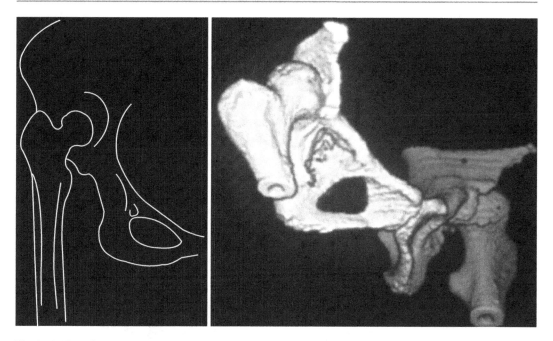

Fig. 3.13 Type C (high dislocation). The femoral head is migrated superiorly and posteriorly to the hypoplastic true acetabulum

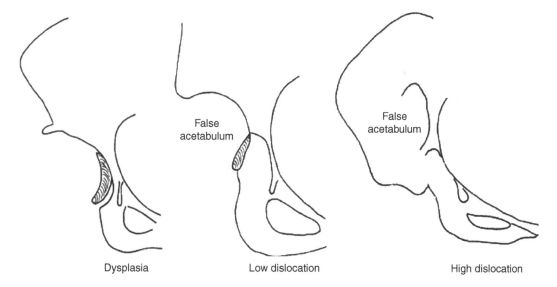

Fig. 3.14 Drawing of the acetabulum in the three types of CHD

Crowe's type III hips and high dislocation corresponds to Crowe's IV hips (Table 3.2) [22].

The requirement of a radiograph of the whole pelvis and the variability of locating the head-neck junction with rotation of the limb are limitations of the Crowe et al. classification. The limitation of Hartofilakidis et al. classification is the difficulty in classifying borderline cases (Figs. 3.18 and 3.19).

The Eftekhar classification recognises four types: dysplasia, intermediate dislocation, high dislocation and old, unreduced dislocation [23]. The Kerboull classification considers the deformity as anterior, intermediate and posterior [20].

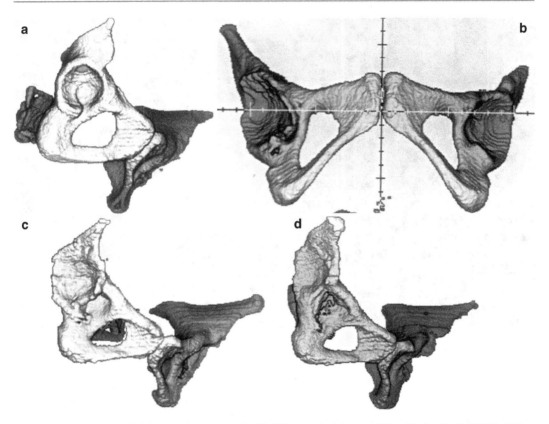

Fig. 3.15 The anatomy of the acetabulum as seen in 3D-CT scans, in (**a**) normal hip, (**b**) dysplastic (*right*), (**c**) low dislocation and (**d**) high dislocation

The inter- and intraobserver reliability of the Crowe and Hartofilakidis classification systems were considered in different studies which concluded that both systems are acceptable because of their high reliability. They offer good to excellent reproducibility and can be used with confidence [24–26].

Interobserver reliability is measured by comparing the ratings of all observers on each occasion, while intraobserver reliability is determined by comparing two assessments of the same observer assessed at different times.

A system is reliable according to the extent of the agreement between repeated measurements [27]. However, for a classification system to be valid, in addition to reliability, it should predict structural bone deformities that are found intraoperatively, thus adding to the treatment planning. A valid classification reveals the underlying

pathology of the disease. It is the best approximation to the "truth" [28, 29]. As stated by Decking et al. [24], if a classification could provide information beyond the simple type of the defect, it would be of superior clinical value.

Reliability and validity are not independent, but are related [30]. However, a classification system may be reliable but not valid, but cannot be valid without being reliable [28]. The Hartofilakidis et al. classification predicting the bone deficiencies encountered during THR, from preoperative radiographs in a reliable and reproducible manner, confirms the validity of the method [31].

To facilitate classification of borderline cases between low dislocation and dysplasia (Fig. 3.18) and between low and high dislocation (Fig. 3.19), we refined our classification system by dividing types B and C in two subtypes with distinct

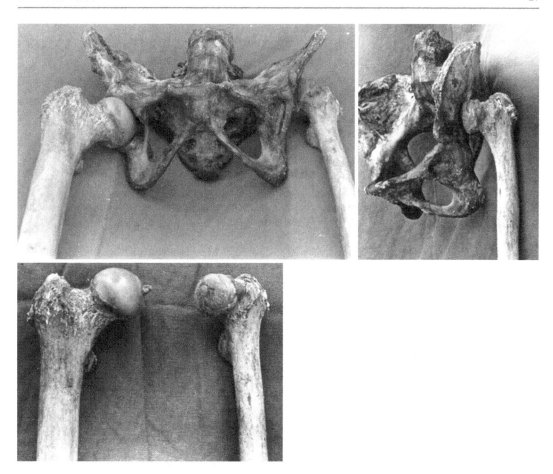

Fig. 3.16 Images illustrate the femur in a cadaveric specimen with high dislocation of the left hip

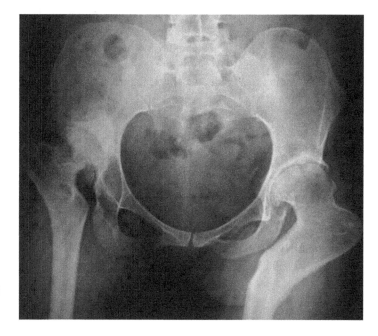

Fig. 3.17 Previous Schanz osteotomies, in this case, with great displacement make THR more challenging

Table 3.2 Description of the Crowe and Hartofilakidis classification systems of congenital hip disease in adults

Classification	Type	Description	Anatomy of the acetabulum as verified during surgery
Crowe et al.	I	Proximal displacement <10 % of pelvic height or less than 50 % subluxation	
	II	Displacement of 10–15 % or subluxation 50–75 %	
	III	Displacement of 15–20 % or subluxation 75–100 %	
	IV	Displacement >20 % or subluxation >100 %	
Hartofilakidis et al.	Dysplasia	The femoral head is contained within the original acetabulum despite the degree of subluxation	Segmental deficiency of the superior wall Secondary shallowness due to fossa-covering osteophyte
	Low dislocation	The femoral head articulates with a false acetabulum which partially covers the true acetabulum to a varying degree	Complete absence of the superior wall Anterior and posterior segmental deficiency Narrow opening and inadequate depth of the true acetabulum
	High dislocation	The femoral head is completely out of the true acetabulum and migrated superiorly and posteriorly to a varying degree	Segmental deficiency of the entire acetabulum with narrow opening Inadequate depth Excessive anteversion Abnormal distribution of bone stock, mainly located superoposteriorly in relation to the true acetabulum

morphological variations each [32]. In the B1 subtype of low dislocation, there is extended cover of the true acetabulum by the false acetabulum, and in the B2 subtype, there is limited cover (Figs. 3.20 and 3.21). In the C1 subtype of high dislocation, there is a false acetabulum high on the iliac wing, and in the C2 subtype, the femoral head lies within the abductor musculature (Fig. 3.22) (Table 3.3) [32].

Xu et al. noticed that the presence or absence of a false acetabulum in high dislocated hips is associated with different loading patterns influencing the development and shape of the proximal femur [33]. They also noticed that the canal width in the proximal part of the femur is much narrowed and more stovepipe shape in type C2 than in type C1, and they suggested that these morphological variations may require different surgical techniques and different implants to reconstruct these hips.

We investigated the possibility of differences following THR in 49 hips of C1 and 30 hips of C2 type, with minimum follow-up of 15 years (15–33). Statistically significant differences were noted in the survival rate ($p=0.001$), leg-lengthening obtained ($p=0.001$) and femoral shortening needed during surgery ($p=0.006$). We concluded that in reporting THR's results in patients with high dislocation, mixing results of two subtypes may lead to statistical bias [34].

In our days, the use of 3D-CT scan allowing the anatomical depiction of the hip facilitates the classification and the preoperative planning and allows for better reconstruction when a THR is decided. It is recommended by the authors in borderline cases.

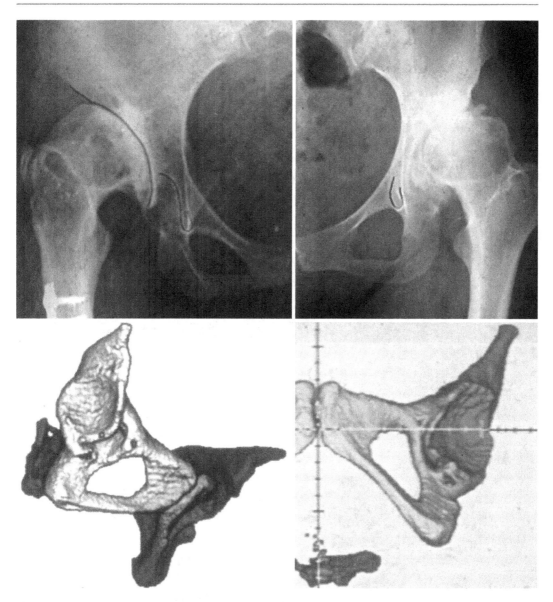

Fig. 3.18 Images illustrate borderline cases of low dislocation (*right hip*) and dysplasia (*left hip*). The 3D-CT scans help the classification of these two hips

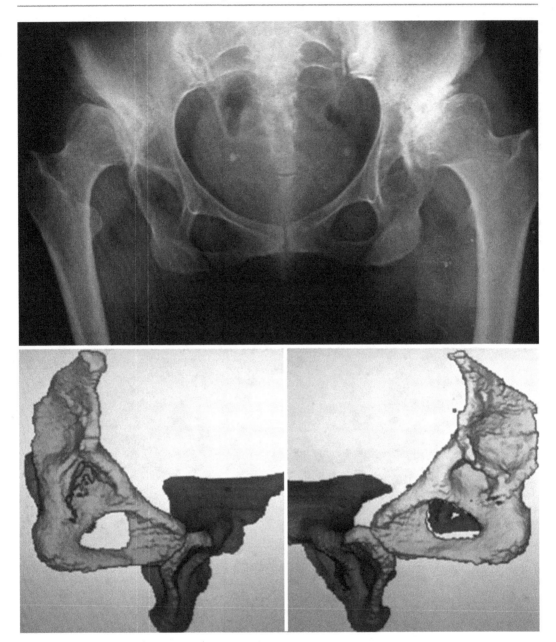

Fig. 3.19 Image illustrates a borderline case of high dislocation (*right hip*) and low dislocation (*left hip*). The need of a 3D-CT scan is obvious

Fig. 3.20 Diagram of the B1 and B2 subtypes of low dislocation

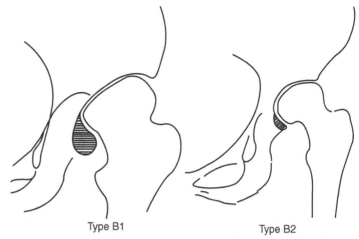

Type B1   Type B2

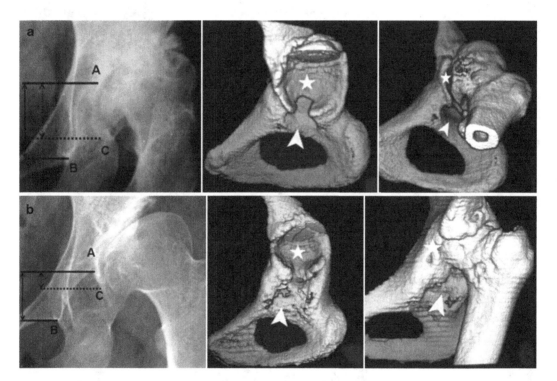

Fig. 3.21 Images illustrate the two subtypes of low dislocation, (**a**) B1 and (**b**) B2. Three points must be recognised on radiographs: (*A*) the superior limit of the true acetabulum; (*B*) the inferior point of the teardrop and (*C*) the most inferior point of the false acetabulum. In 3D-CT scans, *asterisks* depict false acetabulum and *arrowheads* true acetabulum

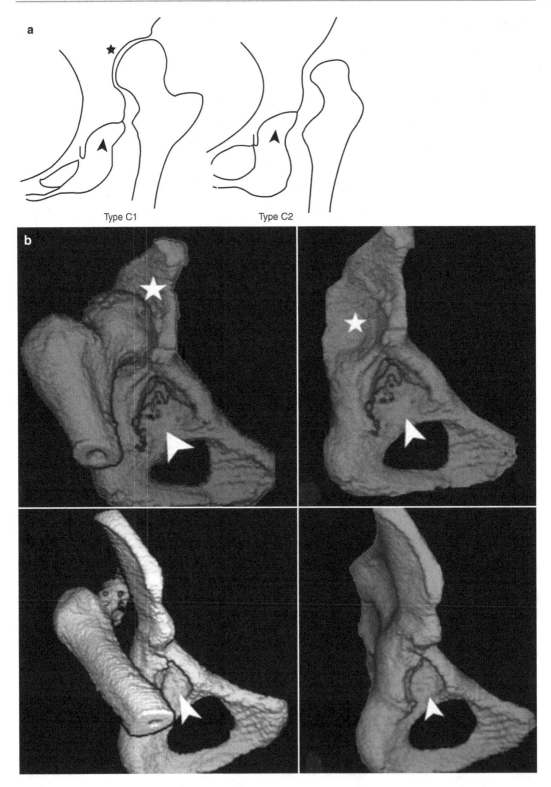

Fig. 3.22 Images illustrate the two subtypes, C1 and C2 of high dislocation. (**a**) Diagram of the two subtypes: C1 when false acetabulum is present and C2 in the absence of a false acetabulum, (**b**) 3D-CT scans of the two subtypes. *Arrowheads* indicate the true and *asterisks* the false acetabulum

Table 3.3 Description of the Hartofilakidis et al. classification system for congenital hip disease in adults and morphological variations of low and high dislocation

CHD type	Description	Subtypes
Dysplasia	The femoral head is contained within the original acetabulum despite the degree of subluxation	A
Low dislocation	The femoral head articulates with a false acetabulum that partially covers the true acetabulum to a varying degree	B1 The false acetabulum covers more than 50 % of the true acetabulum; resembles dysplasia B2 The false acetabulum covers less than 50 % of the true acetabulum; resembles high dislocation
High dislocation	The femoral head is completely out of the true acetabulum and migrated superiorly and posteriorly to a varying degree	C1 The femoral head articulates with a false acetabulum C2 No false acetabulum; the femoral head is free-floating within the gluteal musculature

References

1. Woolacott NF, Puhan MA, Steurer J, Kleijnen J (2005) Ultrasonography in screening for developmental dysplasia of the hip in newborns: systematic review. BMJ 330(7505):1413
2. Hartofilakidis G, Karachalios T, Stamos KG (2000) Epidemiology, demographics, and natural history of congenital hip disease in adults. Orthopedics 23(8):823–827
3. Ganz R, Leunig M, Leunig-Ganz K, Harris WH (2008) The etiology of osteoarthritis of the hip: an integrated mechanical concept. Clin Orthop Relat Res 466(2):264–272
4. Hartofilakidis G, Bardakos NV, Babis GC, Georgiades G (2011) An examination of the association between different morphotypes of femoroacetabular impingement in asymptomatic subjects and the development of osteoarthritis of the hip. J Bone Joint Surg Br 93(5):580–586
5. Roidis NT, Pollalis A, Hartofilakidis G (2013) Total hip arthroplasty in young females with congenital dislocation of the hip, radically improves their long-term quality of life. J Arthroplasty 28(7):1206–1211
6. Dupuytren G (1964) The classic: original or congenital displacement of the head of thigh-bones. Clin Orthop Relat Res 33:3–9
7. Phelps AM (2008) The classic: congenital dislocation of the hip, 1891. Clin Orthop Relat Res 466(4):764–770
8. Dunn PM (1976) The anatomy and pathology of congenital dislocation of the hip. Clin Orthop Relat Res 119:23–27
9. Howorth MB (1947) Congenital dislocation of the hip. Ann Surg 125(2):216–236
10. Howorth MB, Smith HW (1932) Congenital dislocation of the hip treated by open reduction. J Bone Joint Surg Am 12:299–313
11. Massie WK, Howorth MB (1951) Congenital dislocation of the hip. III. Pathogenesis. J Bone Joint Surg Am 33(A:1):190–198
12. Ortolani M (1976) Congenital hip dysplasia in the light of early and very early diagnosis. Clin Orthop Relat Res 119:6–10
13. Stanisavljevic S, Mitchell CL (1963) Congenital dysplasia, subluxation, and dislocation of the hip in stillborn and newborn infants. J Bone Joint Surg Am 45:1147–1158
14. Klisic PJ (1989) Congenital dislocation of the hip–a misleading term: brief report. J Bone Joint Surg Br 71(1):136
15. Hartofilakidis G, Babis GC (2009) Congenital disease of the hip. Clin Orthop Relat Res 467(2):578–579, discussion 580-571
16. Crowe JF, Mani VJ, Ranawat CS (1979) Total hip replacement in congenital dislocation and dysplasia of the hip. J Bone Joint Surg Am 61(1):15–23
17. Hartofilakidis G, Stamos K, Ioannidis TT (1988) Low friction arthroplasty for old untreated congenital dislocation of the hip. J Bone Joint Surg Br 70(2):182–186
18. Hartofilakidis G, Stamos K, Karachalios T, Ioannidis TT, Zacharakis N (1996) Congenital hip disease in adults. Classification of acetabular deficiencies and operative treatment with acetabuloplasty combined with total hip arthroplasty. J Bone Joint Surg Am 78(5):683–692
19. Eftekhar NS (1978) Variations in technique and specific considerations. In: Eftekhar NS (ed) Principles of total hip arthroplasty. CV Mosby, St. Louis, pp 437–455

20. Kerboull M (1994) Arthroplasties totale de hanche par voie transtrochantérienne: editions techniques. In: Encyclopédie Médico Chirurgicale: techniques Chirurgicales- Orthopédie- Traumatologie. Elsevier, Paris, pp 44–668

21. Karachalios T, Hartofilakidis G (2010) Congenital hip disease in adults: terminology, classification, preoperative planning and management. J Bone Joint Surg Br 92(7):914–921

22. Jaroszynski G, Woodgate IG, Saleh KJ, Gross AE (2001) Total hip replacement for the dislocated hip. Instr Course Lect 50:307–316

23. Eftekar NS (1978) Variations in technique and specific considerations. In: Eftekar NS (ed) Principles of total hip arthroplasty. CV Mosby, St. Louis, pp 437–455

24. Decking R, Brunner A, Decking J, Puhl W, Gunther KP (2006) Reliability of the Crowe und Hartofilakidis classifications used in the assessment of the adult dysplastic hip. Skeletal Radiol 35(5):282–287

25. Kose O, Celiktas M, Guler F, Baz AB, Togrul E, Akalin S (2012) Inter- and intraobserver reliability of the Crowe and Hartofilakidis classifications in the assessment of developmental dysplasia of the hip in adult patients. Arch Orthop Trauma Surg 132(11):1625–1630

26. Yiannakopoulos CK, Chougle A, Eskelinen A, Hodgkinson JP, Hartofilakidis G (2008) Inter- and intra-observer variability of the Crowe and Hartofilakidis classification systems for congenital hip disease in adults. J Bone Joint Surg Br 90(5):579–583

27. Garbuz DS, Masri BA, Esdaile J, Duncan CP (2002) Classification systems in orthopaedics. J Am Acad Orthop Surg 10(4):290–297

28. Greenfield ML, Kuhn JE, Wojtys EM (1998) A statistics primer. Validity and reliability. Am J Sports Med 26(3):483–485

29. Kocher MS, Zurakowski D (2004) Clinical epidemiology and biostatistics: a primer for orthopaedic surgeons. J Bone Joint Surg Am 86-A(3):607–620

30. Svanholm H, Starklint H, Gundersen HJ, Fabricius J, Barlebo H, Olsen S (1989) Reproducibility of histomorphologic diagnoses with special reference to the kappa statistic. APMIS 97(8):689–698

31. Yiannakopoulos CK, Xenakis T, Karachalios T, Babis GC, Hartofilakidis G (2009) Reliability and validity of the Hartofilakidis classification system of congenital hip disease in adults. Int Orthop 33(2): 353–358

32. Hartofilakidis G, Yiannakopoulos CK, Babis GC (2008) The morphologic variations of low and high hip dislocation. Clin Orthop Relat Res 466(4):820–824

33. Xu H, Zhou Y, Liu Q, Tang Q, Yin J (2010) Femoral morphologic differences in subtypes of high developmental dislocation of the hip. Clin Orthop Relat Res 468(12):3371–3376

34. Hartofilakidis G, Babis GC, Lampropoulou-Adamidou K, Vlamis J (2013) Results of total hip arthroplasty differ in subtypes of high dislocation. Clin Orthop Relat Res 471(9):2972–2979

Epidemiology, Demographics and Natural History

4

4.1 Epidemiology and Demographics

The reported incidence of neonatal hip dislocation was found to be about 1–2 per 1,000 births [1], and this of neonatal hip instability is higher, between 1.6 and 28.5 per 1,000 [2]. Risk factors are family history, firstborn, breech position, possibly high birth weight and older maternal age as well as swaddling. The latter is considered that exerts unfavourable effect on the future course of an unstable hip [1]. It has been reported that usually instability is transient and resolves spontaneously in the first weeks of life [3].

The published epidemiological data regarding congenital hip disease (CHD) are heterogeneous, due to different diagnostic tools (e.g. physical examination, ultrasonography and plain radiographs), different population's age, different ethnicities/races and geographic location, different observers and the rarity of the disease. Also there is difficulty in distinguishing the neonatal hip dysplasia from the hip instability, which resolves spontaneously. In a study from New Zealand, clinical examination of 20,657 newborns revealed that the 3.2 % were considered to have hip instability at birth. The half of these hips were stabilised completely within 5 days [4].

The incidence of CHD presents significant variability between and within racial groups and geographic locations. Caucasian infants demonstrate 42.2 ‰ (3.8–103 ‰) incidence at birth [1]. Particularly, Sweden has an incidence of 7.6 ‰ [5], England 66.0 ‰ [6], Greece 10.6 ‰ [7] and Italy 6.3 ‰ [8]. Turks, which are Indo-Mediterraneans, have 47.1 ‰ [9], and Africans, in many studies, 0 ‰ [10]. The prevalence is higher in Asians, as Japanese women have 116 ‰ and men 51 ‰ [11]. Differences may be found between residents of the same geographic area with different ethnicities, as the incidence of CHD of general Israeli population is 55 ‰ and that of Ethiopian Jews is much lower (12.4 ‰) [12].

In adults, most epidemiological studies of CHD are based on coincidental urograms or colon radiographs. Percentages vary in the literature depending on the criteria of assessment and the available data used in each study. In adults, the prevalence of CHD is reported to be between 4 and 10 %, which is much higher of that found in newborns may be due to many undiagnosed or subtle cases at birth [13]. The major concern is that CHD is a significant risk factor for the development of secondary osteoarthritis (OA). Radiographic evaluation of 468 patients (660 hips) with OA of the hip of our registry confirmed that 356 hips (54 %) had OA secondary to CHD, 272 hips (41 %) had idiopathic OA and in 74 hips (5 %), the cause of OA was uncertain (Fig. 4.1). In the majority of patients with CHD, both hips are involved. In our registry of the 231 patients with CHD, 125 had bilateral CHD, 17 had idiopathic OA of the contralateral hip and 89 patients had a normal contralateral hip [14].

Among the three types of the disease, dysplasia was found to be more common, while

G. Hartofilakidis et al., *Congenital Hip Disease in Adults*,
DOI 10.1007/978-88-470-5492-9_4, © Springer-Verlag Italia 2014

low and high dislocation were found to have similar incidence. Left and right hips were equally involved in dysplasia and low dislocation, while left-to-right hip ratio was approximately 2:1 in high dislocation. The great majority of patients with CHD (approximately 90 %) were women [14].

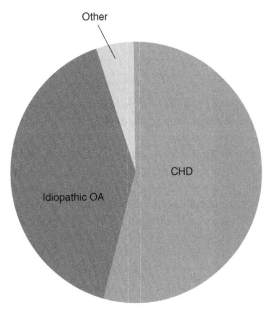

Fig. 4.1 Depiction of the proportion of different types of OA in 660 hips of our registry

4.2   Natural History

Three radiographic types of CHD in infants have been recognised: (1) dysplasia, in which poor acetabular and femoral head development, with an intact Shenton's line, is found, (2) subluxation, in which the Shenton's line is broken, due to the proximal migration of the femoral head, without later overpassing the upper edge of the acetabulum and (3) complete dislocation, in which the femoral head is completely out of the acetabulum [15]. These three types correspond to dysplasia, low dislocation and high dislocation in adults (Table 4.1, Fig. 4.2)

Early diagnosed dysplastic hips are treated successfully with the use for a few months of abduction devices (Figs. 4.3, 4.4 and 4.5). However, the majority of dysplastic hips remain undiagnosed. Diagnosis in these cases is established with the onset of early symptoms usually during the second or third decade of patient's life or as incidental radiographic finding. Dysfunction,

Table 4.1 Congenital hip disease in infants and in adults

Infants	Adults
Dysplasia	Dysplasia
Subluxation	Low dislocation
Dislocation	High dislocation

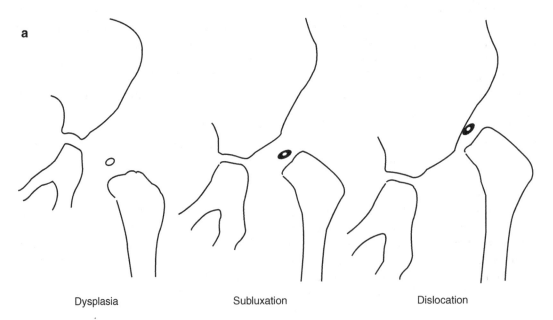

Fig. 4.2 The three types of the disease in infants (**a**) and in adults (**b**)

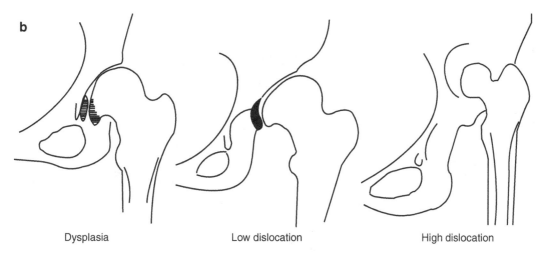

Dysplasia   Low dislocation   High dislocation

Fig. 4.2 (continued)

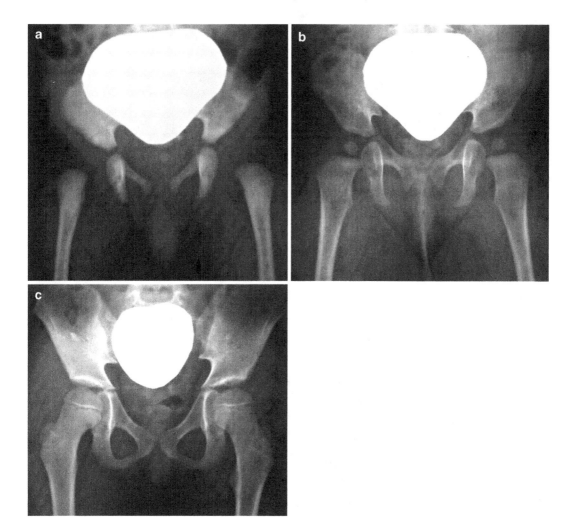

Fig. 4.3 The evolution of dysplastic hips early detected because of family history of CHD. (**a**) The infant's pelvic radiograph 10 days after birth. The inclination of both acetabuli was considered as abnormal and an abduction pillow was applied. (**b**) At the age of 8 months, anteroposterior pelvis radiograph showed normal evolution of the hips and application of the pillow was discontinued. (**c**) Patient at the age of 9 with normal hips

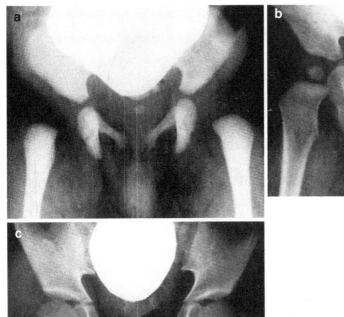

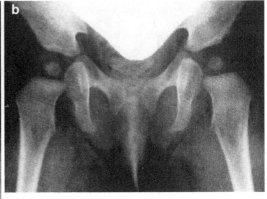

Fig. 4.4 Female with bilateral dysplastic hips. The reason that radiograph was taken in this baby was that her mother was treated by us for bilateral CHD. (**a**) At the age of 3 months. Note the inclination of both acetabuli. An abduction pillow was applied. (**b**) At the age of 13 months, there is normal development of the femoral heads and acetabuli. (**c**) At the latest follow-up, at the age of 8

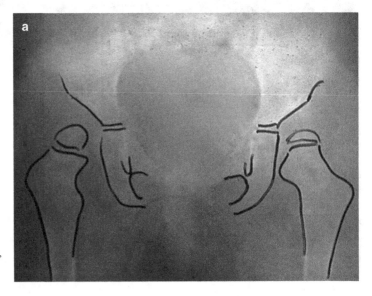

Fig. 4.5 Late diagnosis of dysplastic hips. (**a**) At the age of 3 when the child was first seen by its physician. An abduction frame was applied for 6 months. (**b**) At the age of 35, patient had the first symptoms, pain and limping, due to the development of secondary OA

Fig. 4.5 (continued)

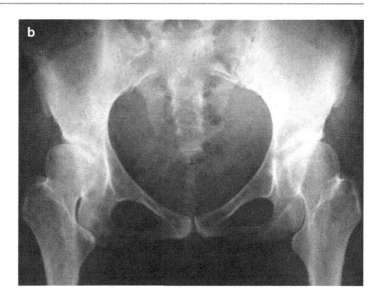

Fig. 4.6 Diagram illustrate the four radiographic indices indicating a normal hip: *WBC* Weight bearing surface (normal value, ±8°), *AA* Acetabular angle (normal value, 25–40°), *CE* Central-edge angle of Wiberg (normal value, 20–40°), *NS* Neck-shaft angle (normal value, 128–135°)

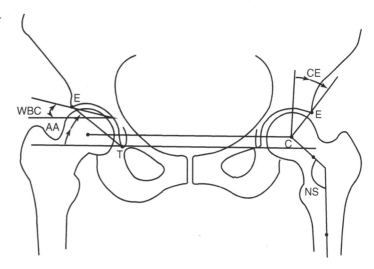

moderate pain and mild limp are the initial symptoms. The definition of a hip as dysplastic is of great importance. In a study, performed on 95 OA-free hips, we found that minor deviation of radiographic indices considered as normal should not characterise a hip as dysplastic and predict the development of OA [16]. The considered as normal values of the four more stated radiographic indices are presented in Fig. 4.6. Degenerative changes in a dysplastic hip develop progressively following biomechanical patterns (Fig. 4.7) [17–19]. The superolateral joint space gradually narrows and the femoral head becomes elliptical, due to the formation of marginal osteophytes.

At this final stage, pain and limping become more severe. Large cysts, both in the acetabulum and femoral head, are formed and subluxation is increased.

Untreated patients with subluxation are limping since infancy, but pain usually starts later, at the age of 25–30 years. Degenerative changes develop within the false acetabulum, following the same biomechanical patterns as in the dysplastic hips (Figs. 4.8, 4.9 and 4.10).

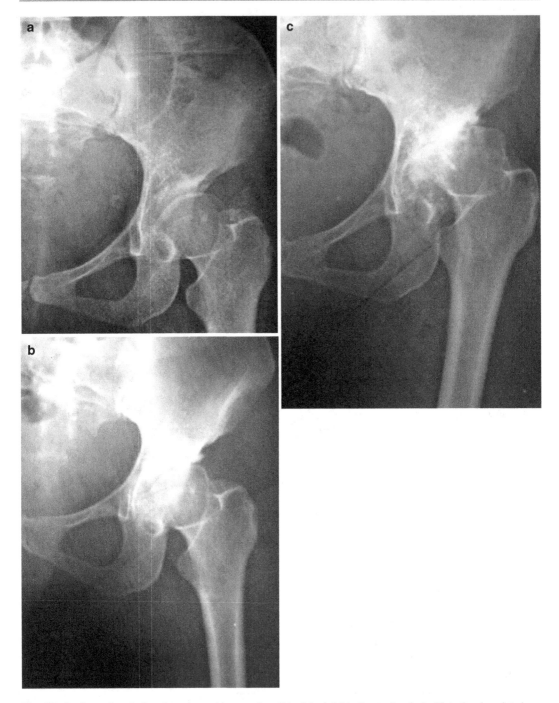

Fig. 4.7 Radiographs of a female patient with secondary OA of the left hip due to dysplasia. Note the slow deterioration. (**a**) When the patient was 30 years old. (**b**) At the age of 38. (**c**) At the age of 47 when THR was decided

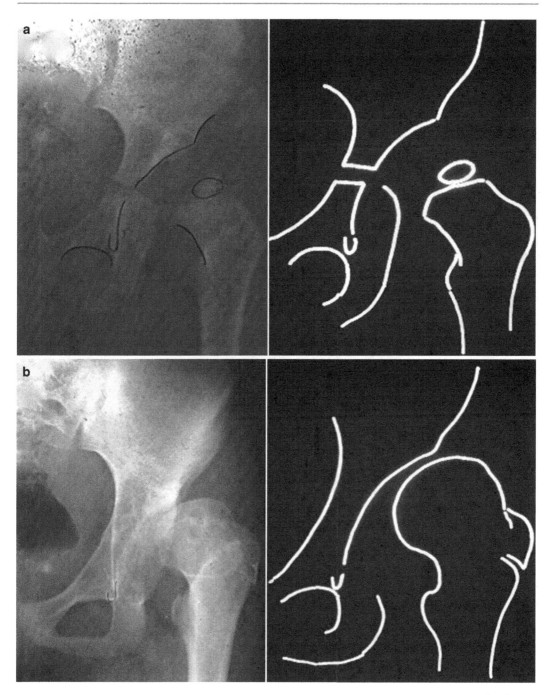

Fig. 4.8 Radiographs and diagrams of a female patient with subluxation of the left hip at infancy developed to low dislocation. (**a**) At the age of 2. (**b**) At the age of 12. (**c**) At the age of 16, after subtrochanteric osteotomy. (**d**) The final image, when the patient was 37 years old

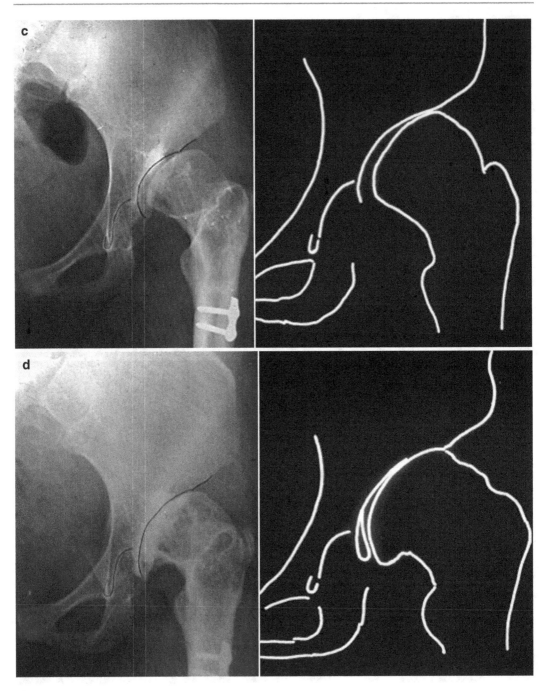

Fig. 4.8 (continued)

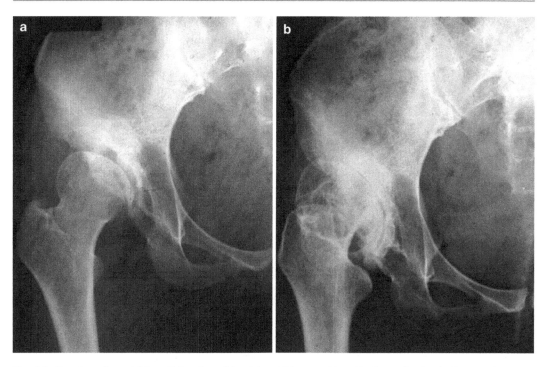

Fig. 4.9 Female patient with low dislocation of the right hip. She was limping since infancy but pain started at the age of approximately 35. (**a**) When the patient was 24 years old and had no pain. (**b**) At the age of 49. Pain was severe and limping worsened. A THR was followed

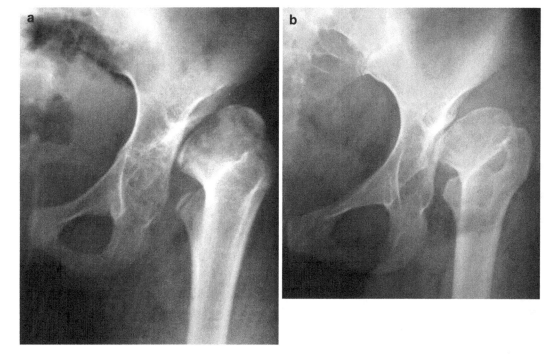

Fig. 4.10 Female with low dislocation at the age of (**a**) 15, (**b**) 26, (**c**) 46 when THR was advised

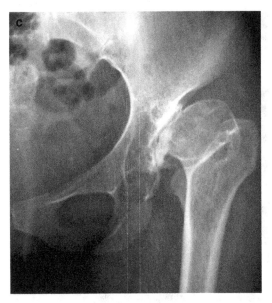

Fig. 4.10 (continued)

The natural history of complete dislocated hips depends, mainly, on two factors: the presence of unilateral or bilateral deformity and whether a false acetabulum is present (Figs. 4.11, 4.12 and 4.13). In unilateral involvement disability generally is greater, and limping and leg-length discrepancy more severe. The patients complain for low-back pain and pain mainly in the ipsilateral knee, which develops a gradually increased valgus deformity and OA. In unilateral cases, thoracolumbar scoliosis is present and in bilateral increased lordosis of the lumbar spine is common. Pain starts at an average of 30 years in hips with a false acetabulum, and much later at the age of 40–45 years in hips without false acetabulum, probably due to muscle fatigue.

The natural history of all three types can be potentially altered by previous treatments (Figs. 4.14, 4.15 and 4.16). Knowledge of

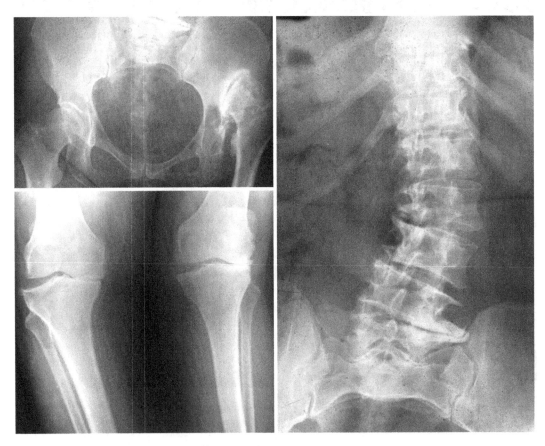

Fig. 4.11 Images illustrate the case of a female patient, 60 years old, with unilateral high dislocation. Delay of surgical intervention led to severe spine and both knee deformities (ipsilateral valgus with OA of the lateral compartment and contralateral varus with OA of the medial compartment)

Fig. 4.12 Images illustrate the case of a female patient with bilateral high dislocation. (**a**) Radiograph at the age of 2. Unsuccessful treatment was applied. (**b**) Radiograph at the age of 33 when the patient was consulted for bilateral THRs

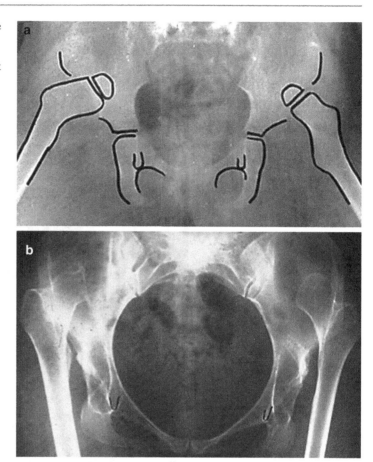

the natural history of CHD facilitates the understanding of the potential development and progress of the disease, which differs among the three types. It can lead to a better understanding of the anatomical abnormalities found in the different types and thus facilitates preoperative planning and choice of the most appropriate therapeutic measures for adult patients [14].

Fig. 4.13 Images illustrate the case of a female patient with bilateral high dislocation. (**a**) At the age of 20. (**b**) At the age of 40, painful OA was developed on the right hip with the false acetabulum

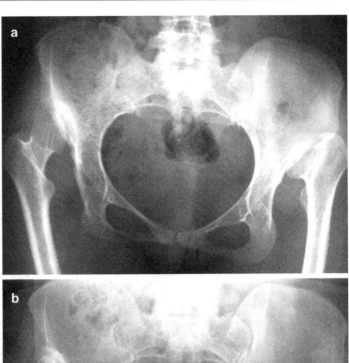

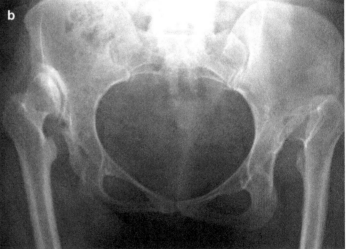

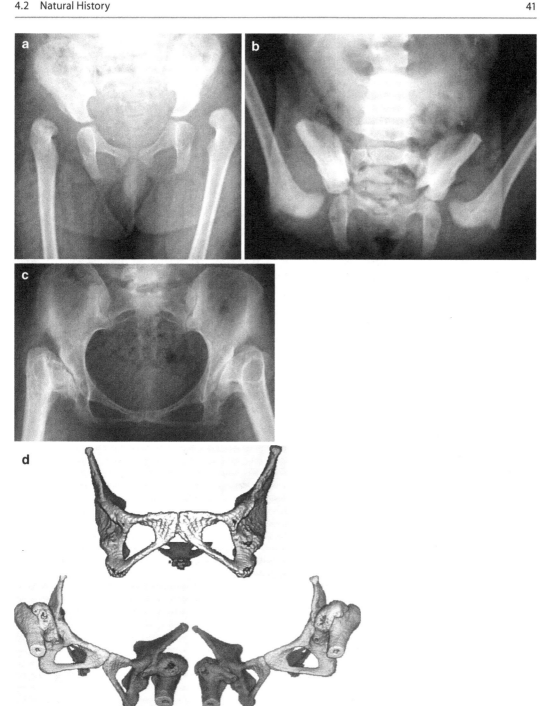

Fig. 4.14 Images illustrate the case of a female patient born with bilateral complete dislocation. (**a**) At the age of one. (**b**) Reduction and immobilisation in plaster for 8 months. Note the extreme abduction in which the hips were immobilised. Open reduction of both hips was followed. (**c**) Radiograph taken when the patient referred to us, at the age of 28. Severe damage of both femoral head epiphyses. (**d**) 3D-CT scans illustrate the extent of the deformity bilaterally

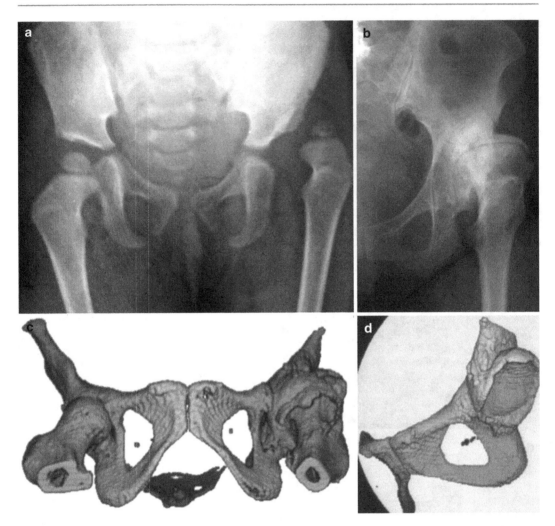

Fig. 4.15 Images illustrate the case of a patient with left completely dislocated hip. (**a**) Radiograph taken at the age of 2. As referred to patient's record, unsuccessful conservative treatment was applied. (**b**) At the age of 43, severe secondary OA had developed. (**c, d**) 3D-CT scans demonstrate the anatomy of the hip with and without the femoral head

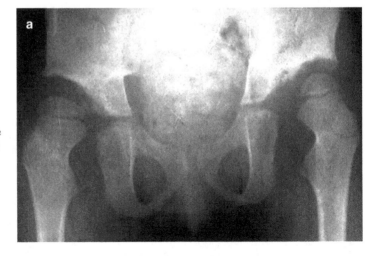

Fig. 4.16 Images illustrate the case of a female patient with subluxation of both hips. (**a**) At the age of 4, 1 year after Chiari osteotomy bilaterally. Hips remained subluxated. (**b**) At the age of 36, when the patient was examined by us, both hips presented low dislocation with secondary OA

Fig. 4.16 (continued)

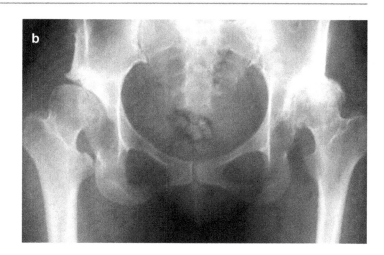

References

1. Loder TL, Skopelja EN (2011) The epidemiology and demographics of hip dysplasia. ISRN Orthop 46
2. Leck I (2000) Congenital dislocation of the hip. In: Wald N, Leck I (eds) Antenatal and neonatal screening, 2nd edn. Oxford University Press, Oxford, pp 398–424
3. Dezateux C, Rosendahl K (2007) Developmental dysplasia of the hip. Lancet 369(9572):1541–1552
4. Hadlow V (1988) Neonatal screening for congenital dislocation of the hip. A prospective 21-year survey. J Bone Joint Surg Br 70(5):740–743
5. Danielsson LG (2000) Instability of the hip in neonates. An ethnic and geographical study in 24,101 newborn infants in Malmo. J Bone Joint Surg Br 82(4):545–547
6. Bache CE, Clegg J, Herron M (2002) Risk factors for developmental dysplasia of the hip: ultrasonographic findings in the neonatal period. J Pediatr Orthop B 11(3):212–218
7. Giannakopoulou C, Aligizakis A, Korakaki E, Velivasakis E, Hatzidaki E, Manoura A, Bakataki A, Hadjipavlou A (2002) Neonatal screening for developmental dysplasia of the hip on the maternity wards in Crete. Greece. Correlation to risk factors. Clin Exp Obstet Gynecol 29(2):148–152
8. Riboni G, Bellini A, Serantoni S, Rognoni E, Bisanti L (2003) Ultrasound screening for developmental dysplasia of the hip. Pediatr Radiol 33(7): 475–481
9. Dogruel H, Atalar H, Yavuz OY, Sayli U (2008) Clinical examination versus ultrasonography in detecting developmental dysplasia of the hip. Int Orthop 32(3):415–419
10. Poul J, Garvie D, Grahame R, Saunders AJ (1998) Ultrasound examination of neonate's hip joints. J Pediatr Orthop B 7(1):59–61
11. Inoue K, Wicart P, Kawasaki T, Huang J, Ushiyama T, Hukuda S, Courpied J (2000) Prevalence of hip osteoarthritis and acetabular dysplasia in french and japanese adults. Rheumatology (Oxford) 39(7):745–748
12. Eidelman M, Chezar A, Bialik V (2002) Developmental dysplasia of the hip incidence in Ethiopian Jews revisited: 7-year prospective study. J Pediatr Orthop B 11(4):290–292
13. Jacobsen S (2006) Adult hip dysplasia and osteoarthritis. Studies in radiology and clinical epidemiology. Acta Orthop Suppl 77(324):1–37
14. Hartofilakidis G, Karachalios T, Stamos KG (2000) Epidemiology, demographics, and natural history of congenital hip disease in adults. Orthopedics 23(8): 823–827
15. Weinstein SL (1987) Natural history of congenital hip dislocation (CDH) and hip dysplasia. Clin Orthop Relat Res 225:62–76
16. Vossinakis IC, Georgiades G, Kafidas D, Hartofilakidis G (2008) Unilateral hip osteoarthritis: can we predict the outcome of the other hip? Skeletal Radiol 37(10): 911–916. doi:10.1007/s00256-008-0522-8
17. Pauwels F (1984) Biomechanical principles of varus/valgus intertrochanteric osteotomy in the treatment of osteoarthritis of the hip. In: Schatzker J (ed) The intertrochanteric osteotomy. Springer, Berlin, pp 3–23
18. Bombelli R (1976) Osteoarthritis of the hip: pathogenesis and consequent. Springer, Berlin
19. Bombelli R, Aronson J (1984) Biomechanical classification of osteoarthritis of the hip with special reference to treatment techniques and results. In: Schatzker J (ed) The intertrochanteric osteotomy. Springer, Berlin, pp 67–134

Treatment Options, Except Total Hip Replacement: Conservative Management and Osteotomies

5

5.1 Conservative Management

Treatment of secondary osteoarthritis (OA) due to congenital hip disease (CHD) in adults is surgical, when pain and disability of the patients significantly alter their quality of life. Before this stage, non-pharmacological conservative treatment includes education, physiotherapy, weight reduction and avoidance of extreme activities, including sports, except swimming. In older patients, the use of a cane may postpone, for a few years, the need for surgery.

Pharmacological treatment options may include:

- Simple analgesics like paracetamol
- Symptomatic slow-acting drugs in OA (SYSADOA) like hyaluronanic acid, chondroitin sulphate, glucosamine sulphate and diacereine. Their therapeutic role in terms of pain relief and slowing the progression of OA is debated [1].
- Nonsteroidal anti-inflammatory drugs (NSAIDs). Although they are acting immediately to inflammation, which is the main cause of pain in the initial stages of OA, these drugs are associated with serious adverse events particularly from the gastrointestinal system. The development of selective cyclo-oxygenase-2 (COX-2) inhibitors reduces the incidence of upper gastrointestinal tract ulcerations; however, other toxicities such as hypertension, cardiovascular events and thromboembolic complications still remain a considerable risk [2, 3].

- Intra-articular corticosteroids are also used, particularly when there is moderate to severe pain not responding to the above-mentioned oral medications. However, repeated injections are considered harmful for the joint cartilage and are not recommended [4].

To date we can only treat symptoms in mild to moderate cases but we cannot modify the course of the disease. The management of OA is limited to control pain and inflammation. The aim of recent pharmacological studies is the development of conservative treatment of OA with chondroprotective or chondrotherapeutic agents.

5.2 Osteotomies

The treatment of choice in patients with dysplastic hips before the advent of total hip replacement (THR) was intertrochanteric and pelvic osteotomies [5–14]. Pauwels' main concept, expanded by Bombelli, was that the reduction of excessive joint pressure, in dysplastic hips, may prevent the development of OA.

Osteotomies were the only surgical solution, at these early years, and as they were performed without clear indications, their results were not always successful. Best results were obtained, with the varus intertrochanteric osteotomy, in the dysplastic hips at the early stage of the degenerative changes and with the valgus osteotomy at a later stage (Figs. 5.1 and 5.2). The

G. Hartofilakidis et al., *Congenital Hip Disease in Adults*, DOI 10.1007/978-88-470-5492-9_5, © Springer-Verlag Italia 2014

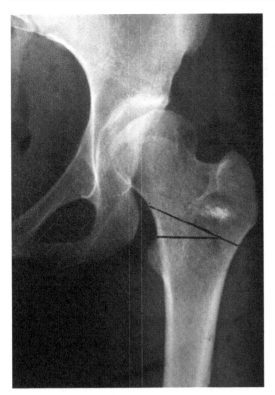

Fig. 5.1 Varus osteotomy performed by removal of a bony wedge with a medial base

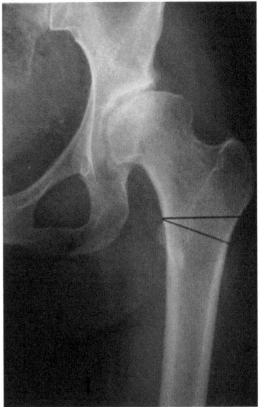

Fig. 5.2 Valgus osteotomy performed by removal of a bony wedge with a lateral base

senior author of this book (GH) used these types of osteotomies, during the 1960s and 1970s with good results (Figs. 5.3, 5.4 and 5.5).

Other types of osteotomies, like McMurray [15] (Fig. 5.6) and Schanz [16] (Fig. 5.7) were also performed in more severe types of CHD.

Pelvic osteotomies used after fusion of the centres of ossification are the rotational (spherical or dial) acetabular [17], the periacetabular [8, 18] and the triple osteotomy [19]. There were no clear indications for the use of each type of pelvic osteotomy and therefore they were used according to the surgeon's preference and/or experience. Pelvic osteotomies were used to reorient the dysplastic acetabulum, thus covering

the femoral head, in cases where the degenerative changes were mild and the femoral head had not lost its congruity with the acetabulum. Some of the complications of the pelvic osteotomies are the intra-articular fractures; injury of great vessels such as the femoral, the obturator and the superior gluteal; injury of nerves, particularly of the femoral as well as technical errors which are not rare and are hardly corrected.

In our days, intertrochanteric and pelvic osteotomies in adults seldom are performed and as surgeons have limited experience in this type of operations should be decided with caution.

Fig. 5.3 Twenty-eight-year-old female with bilateral dysplastic hips. She had mild pain for 2 years of the right hip. In 1983, we performed a varus intertrochanteric osteotomy in both hips within 20 days. (**a**) Preoperative radiograph. (**b**) Thirty years after osteotomies. Patient, at the age of 58, is free of symptoms

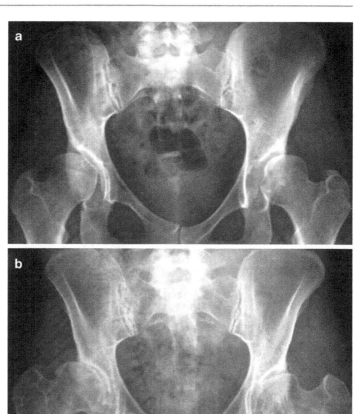

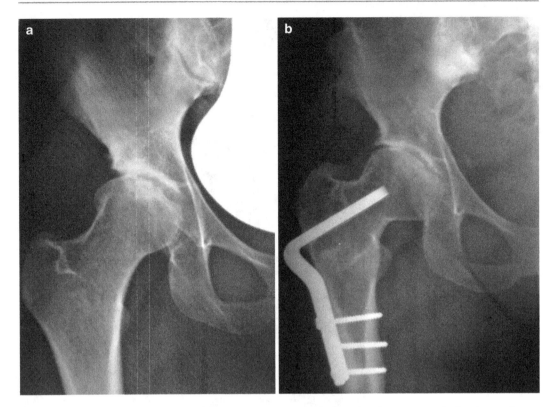

Fig. 5.4 Twenty-three-year-old female with dysplastic right hip. In 1975, we performed a varus intertrochanteric osteotomy. (**a**) Preoperative radiograph. (**b**) Radiograph taken 23 years after the osteotomy. At that time, at the age of 46, she is still free of symptoms

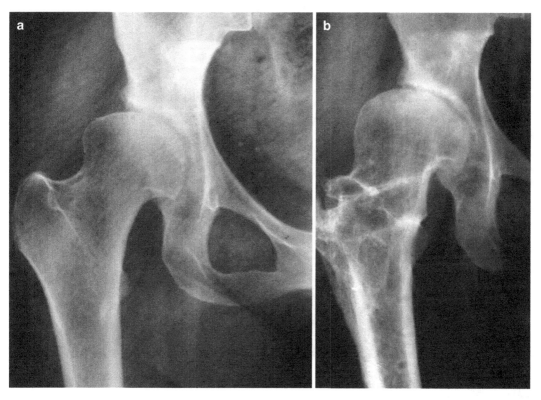

Fig. 5.5 (**a**) Preoperative radiograph of a female patient at the age of 34 with a dysplastic hip at the second stage of evolution of degenerative changes. In 1987, we per-formed a valgus intertrochanteric osteotomy. (**b**) After 17 years, she started having mild pain. Three years later, THR was performed

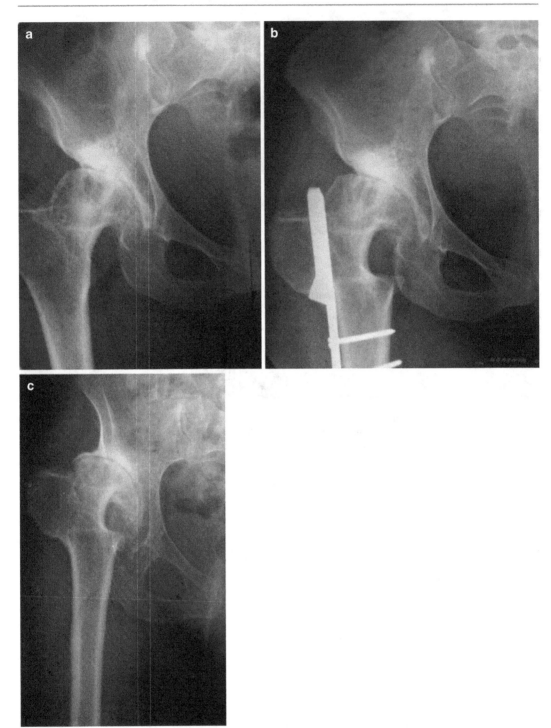

Fig. 5.6 (a) Dysplastic hip of a 30-year-old female. In 1970 a McMurray osteotomy was decided, as the better solution. (b) One year after surgery. (c) Twenty-three years after osteotomy when THR was recommended

Fig. 5.7 (**a**) Female patient at the age of 31 in 1962. She had a dysplastic right hip and a left hip with low dislocation. In 1964, as the only surgical solution at that time, she had a Schanz osteotomy on the left hip and in 1975 a McMurray osteotomy on the right hip. (**b**) Radiograph taken in 1994, when the patient was 63 years old and came to us with severe secondary OA of both hips

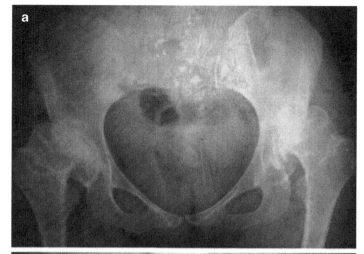

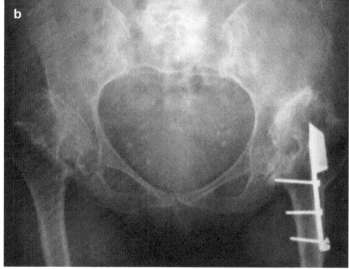

References

1. Bruyere O, Burlet N, Delmas PD, Rizzoli R, Cooper C, Reginster JY (2008) Evaluation of symptomatic slow-acting drugs in osteoarthritis using the GRADE system. BMC Musculoskelet Disord 9:165
2. Sostres C, Gargallo CJ, Arroyo MT, Lanas A (2010) Adverse effects of non-steroidal anti-inflammatory drugs (NSAIDs, aspirin and coxibs) on upper gastrointestinal tract. Best Pract Res Clin Gastroenterol 24(2):121–132
3. Brophy JM (2007) Cardiovascular effects of cyclooxygenase-2 inhibitors. Curr Opin Gastroenterol 23(6):617–624
4. Zhang W, Moskowitz RW, Nuki G, Abramson S, Altman RD, Arden N, Bierma-Zeinstra S, Brandt KD, Croft P, Doherty M, Dougados M, Hochberg M, Hunter DJ, Kwoh K, Lohmander LS, Tugwell P (2008) OARSI recommendations for the management of hip and knee osteoarthritis, part II: OARSI evidence-based, expert consensus guidelines. Osteoarthritis Cartilage 16(2):137–162
5. Pauwels F (1984) Biomechanical principles of varus/valgus intertrochanteric osteotomy in the treatment of osteoarthritis of the hip. In: Schatzker J (ed) The intertrochanteric osteotomy. Springer, Berlin, pp 3–23
6. Bombelli R (1976) Osteoarthritis of the hip: pathogenesis and consequent. Springer, Berlin
7. Bombelli R, Aronson J (1984) Biomechanical classification of osteoarthritis of the hip with special reference to treatment techniques and results. In: Schatzker J (ed) The intertrochanteric osteotomy. Springer, Berlin, pp 67–134
8. Trousdale RT, Ekkernkamp A, Ganz R, Wallrichs SL (1995) Periacetabular and intertrochanteric osteotomy for the treatment of osteoarthrosis in dysplastic hips. J Bone Joint Surg Am 77(1):73–85

9. Pauwels F (1976) Biomechanics of the normal and diseased hip. Springer, Berlin

10. Morscher E, Feinstein R (1984) Results of intertrochanteric osteotomy in the treatment of osteoarthritis of the hip. In: Schatzker J (ed) The intertrochanteric osteotomy. Springer, Berlin, pp 169–179

11. Muller ME (1984) Interochanteric osteotomy: indications, preoperative planning, technique. In: Schatzker J (ed) The intertrochanteric osteotomy. Springer, Berlin, pp 25–67

12. Schneider R (1984) Intertrochanteric osteotomy in osteoarthrtis of the hip joint. In: Schatzker J (ed) The intertrochanteric osteotomy. Springer, Berlin, pp 135–169

13. Poss R (1984) The role of osteotomy in the treatment of osteoarthritis of the hip. J Bone Joint Surg Am 66(1):144–151

14. Millis MB, Poss R, Murphy SB (1992) Osteotomies of the hip in the prevention and treatment of osteoarthritis. Instr Course Lect 41:145–154

15. McMurray TP (1939) Osteo-arthritis of the hip joint. J Bone Joint Surg Am 21(1):1–11

16. Schanz A (1925) Ueber die nach Schenkelhalsbrüchen zurückbleibenden Gehstörungen. Dtsch Med Wochenschr 51:730

17. Wagner H (1978) Experiences with spherical acetabular osteotomy for the correction of the dysplastic acetabulum. Progr Orthop Surg 2:131–145

18. Ganz R, Klaue K, Vinh TS, Mast JW (1988) A new periacetabular osteotomy for the treatment of hip dysplasias. Technique and preliminary results. Clin Orthop Relat Res 232:26–36

19. Tonnis D, Behrens K, Tscharani F (1981) A new technique of triple osteotomy for turning dysplastic acetabula in adolescents and adults (author's transl). Z Orthop Ihre Grenzgeb 119(3):253–265

6

Total Hip Replacement: Indications and Preoperative Assessment

The introduction of total hip replacement (THR) by the pioneers in the field, John Charnley [1] and McKee Farrar [2], radically changed the treatment of congenital hip disease (CHD) in adult patients. The older methods, such as of osteotomies and excision arthroplasties, were gradually abandoned in favour of the new revolutionary method of THR. During the first years, a scepticism existed and even Charnley [3] stated that THR, in some technically difficult cases of high dislocation, should be avoided. However, in the next years, new techniques and implants made THR feasible even in these extreme cases. The last 20–25 years the literature is full of articles reflecting the worldwide experience on the field (see Chap. 8).

THR became an exceptionally significant procedure for the treatment of CHD in adults (Figs. 8.2 and 8.3). However, it may involve unexpected disappointment (Figs. 10.9, 10.10, 10.11 and 10.12). Therefore, it is imperative to be decided when it is absolutely necessary. Orthopaedic surgeons should protect this operation from the overuse. The patients should be informed for the severity of the procedure, for potential complications and that their new artificial joint is a subject of physical wear.

The term "total hip replacement (THR)" than "total hip arthroplasty (THA)" must be used. This term is more accurate because it reminds that this is an irreversible procedure in which the destroyed joint is removed and replaced by an artificial one. "Arthroplasty", a compound Greek word, has the meaning of joint anaplasis/formation and may be misleading for both the surgeon and the patient.

6.1 Indications

Due to surgical difficulties and serious complications of THR in patients with CHD, the operation should be reserved for very selected patients who realise the increased risks and the possibility of failure [4]. Obviously, an experienced surgeon familiar with these hips must perform THR in dislocated hips, and only when there is a clear indication [4]. The simple fact that new methods and prostheses have developed and, also, that our surgical experience has increased are no reasons for early intervention (Fig. 6.1).

Pain and/or severe functional impairment with severe limping, before pelvic inclination, fixed flexion deformity of the hip and knee and spinal deformities have been established are the main indications for surgery. Mild limping alone is not an indication, especially in young active patients. These patients should be encouraged to avoid extreme daily activities and occasionally use anti-inflammatory drugs and follow a programme of adapted physiotherapy (Figs. 6.2 and 6.3) [5].

Age is a factor that should be carefully considered. THR is generally avoided in young patients. However, there are cases where surgery is decided after careful evaluation of patients' symptoms in combination with their psychological status (Fig. 6.4).

According to the authors' experience, patients with different types of CHD present for THR at an average of 35–45 years, depending on the osteoarthritic changes and the coexisting deformities [6]. In many patients surgery can be

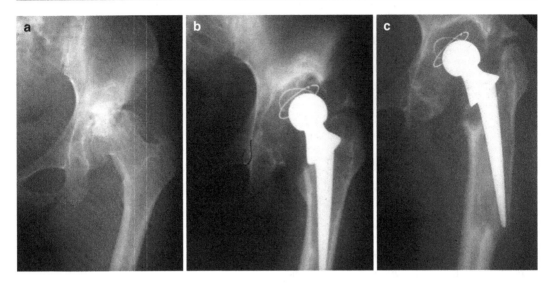

Fig. 6.1 (**a**) This patient with a dysplastic left hip, at the age of 33, had only mild limp without pain. She was operated without clear indications. (**b**) Radiograph one year postoperatively. The cup was not inserted in the right place as the surgeon did not notice in the preopera- tive radiograph that the femoral head was articulated with a false acetabulum and the stem was fixed in varus and penetrated the lateral cortex. (**c**) The hip was revised 7 years later, after incomplete follow-up that resulted in major bone stock loss

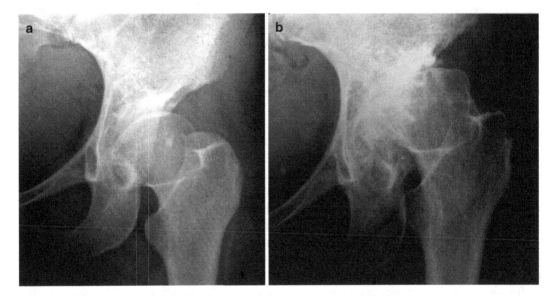

Fig. 6.2 (**a**) This patient at the age of 30 had only mild limp without pain. (**b**) Surgery was postponed for 17 years

delayed for a few or more years. Nonetheless, any adaptive changes as a consequence of a surgery's postponement should be considered, especially those on the knees and the spine (Fig. 6.5). The gold standard is the operation to be decided "not too early, but not too late", and the decision should be taken in consultation with the patient. He must be informed for the benefits as well as for the possible complications and that some limping may persist postoperatively.

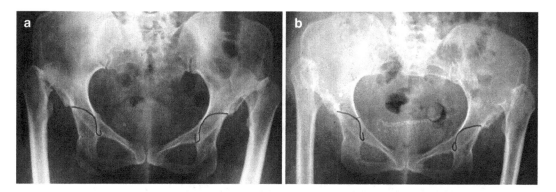

Fig. 6.3 Patient with bilateral high dislocation. (**a**) Operation was postponed at the age of 42 (**b**) to the age of 53, because symptoms were tolerable

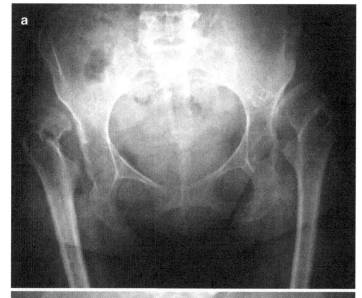

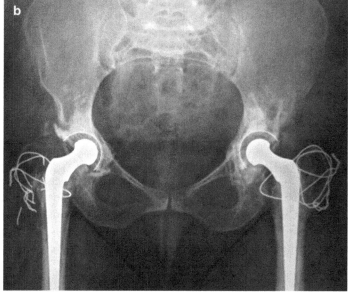

Fig. 6.4 This female patient was only 29 years old when she was first examined. She had heavy limping and was in bad psychological state. She was taken antidepressants and avoided to communicate with others. (**a**) Preoperative radiograph. After many consultations, surgery was decided. (**b**) After bilateral THRs her life changed radically. She married, she has two children and she remains a happy and healthy woman all these 24 years since surgery, enjoying the more productive years of her life

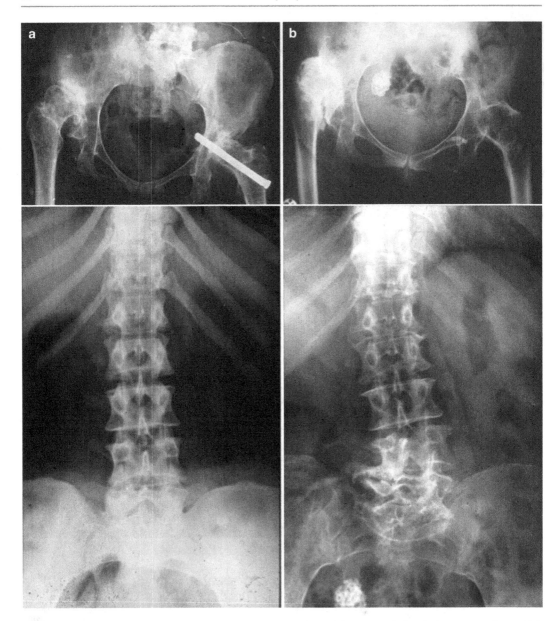

Fig. 6.5 (a) The patient's left hip with dysplasia was fused at the age of 26 in 1956. Right hip, with low dislocation, was left without treatment. (b) For 36 years she was avoiding any medical assistance; as a result her disability was greatly aggravated. Surgical reconstruction, which followed by us, encountered major difficulties and patient's disability remained great due to spinal deformities and degenerative changes

6.2 Preoperative Assessment

Preoperative assessment is recommended in all THRs. In CHD, it is vital to establish the type of the disease and the severity of the deformity. Good-quality radiographs of the pelvis are needed. The extent and location of the segmental defects are estimated, as are the diameter and depth of the acetabulum (useful for the estimation of the required size of the acetabular component), the distribution of bone stock and the anteversion of the acetabulum and the femoral

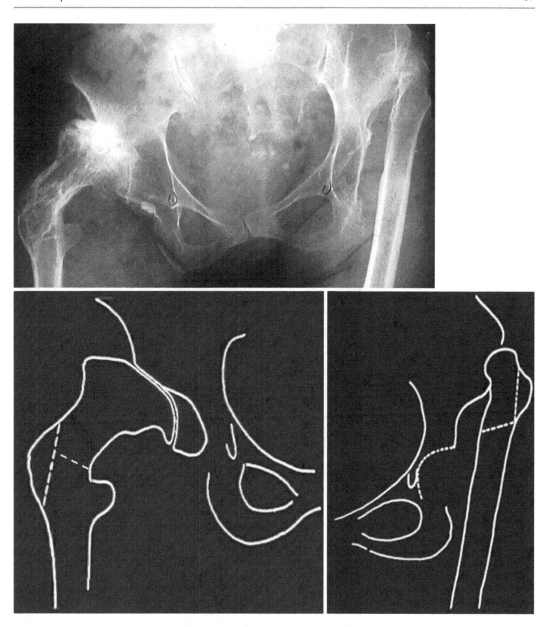

Fig. 6.6 This patient had high dislocation on the left hip and low dislocation on the right with previous varus intertrochanteric osteotomy. Preoperative drawing helps the surgeon to plan the steps to be followed during the operation on both hips

neck. The proximal femur is assessed to estimate the type and size of the femoral component to be used for reconstruction. The surgeon should be informed of the difficulties of the procedure in order to avoid complications and organise the use of the proper technique and implants (Fig. 6.1).

Also, the need of bone grafts is estimated. The availability of special instruments that will be needed during surgery should be ordered and checked. In certain cases it is important to draw the bone cuts and the position of the appropriate implant on the radiograph (Figs. 6.6, 6.7 and 6.8).

Fig. 6.7 (**a**) Preoperative assessment in this case is necessary in order to facilitate the reconstruction of both femurs which were deformed by previous Schanz osteotomies. (**b**) According to planning the right hip could have primary THR by osteotomising the greater trochanter and shortening the femur at the level of femoral neck. The left hip necessitated a corrective osteotomy to align the femoral canal before THR

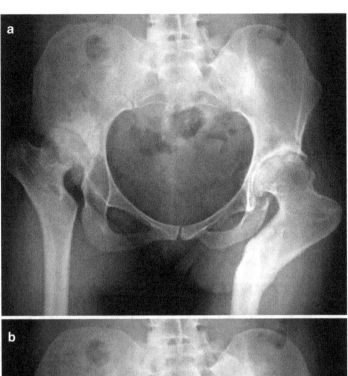

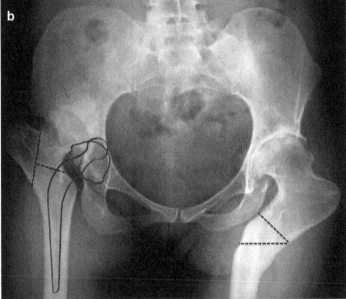

Some surgeons are using templates, both for the assessment of the acetabulum and of the femur, while in borderline cases CT or 3D-CT scans are necessary (Figs. 6.9 and 6.10).

The preoperative height of the dislocation is measured with the method of Crowe as the vertical distance between the lower part of the teardrop and the femoral head-neck junction (Fig. 6.11).

Fig. 6.8 (**a**) A 60-year-old female with high dislocation of the right hip. At the age of 14, in 1949, she had fusion of the joint with the extraarticular method of Brittain [7]. (**b**) Preoperative assessment by drawing the bone cuts and the position of the implants that will be used. The removal of fusion bone bar before any attempt to dislocate the hip joint was necessary to avoid intraoperative fracture

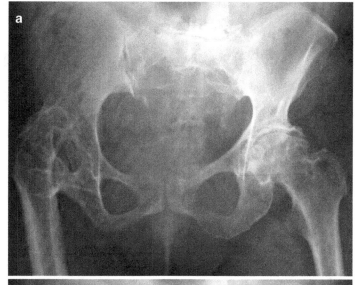

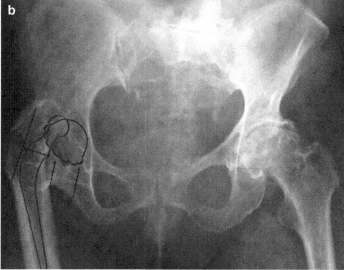

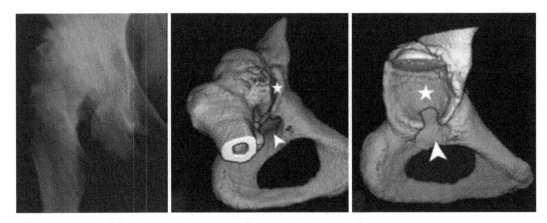

Fig. 6.9 A borderline case between dysplasia and B1 subtype of low dislocation. 3D-CT scan proves that the femoral head is articulated with a false acetabulum (*asterisks*) that covers to a great degree the true acetabulum (*arrow heads*). The case is a B1 subtype of low dislocation. The surgeon should be prepared to look for the true acetabulum underneath the lower part of the false acetabulum

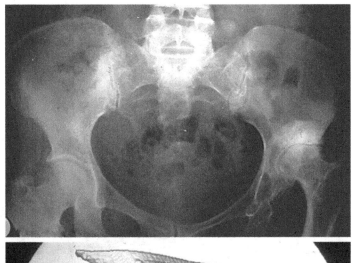

Fig. 6.10 A borderline case between high dislocation and B2 subtype of low dislocation. The answer was given by the performance of a 3D-CT scan which revealed clearly that the case was a B2 low dislocation. This is an important information for the surgeon to be prepared for the technique and implants that will be needed for the reconstruction of the deficient acetabulum

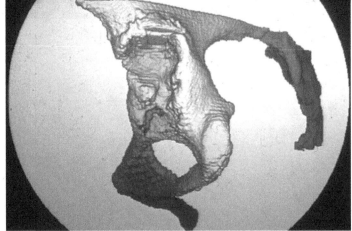

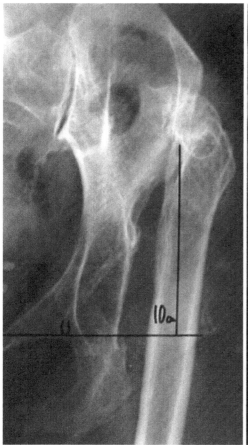 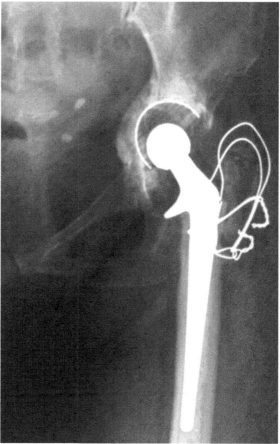

Fig. 6.11 Measurement of the height of the dislocation is crucial for the surgeon to plan this operation. In this case the height of the dislocation was measured 10 cm. Proximal shortening of the femur was needed to be extended to the lower part of the lesser trochanter. (See also Fig. 7.10)

References

1. Charnley J (1961) Arthroplasty of the hip. A new operation. Lancet 1(7187):1129–1132
2. McKee GK, Watson-Farrar J (1966) Replacement of arthritic hips by the McKee-Farrar prosthesis. J Bone Joint Surg Br 48(2):245–259
3. Charnley J, Feagin JA (1973) Low-friction arthroplasty in congenital subluxation of the hip. Clin Orthop Relat Res 91:98–113
4. Eftekhar NS (1993) Congenital displasia and dislocation. Summary of essentials. In: Eftekhar NS (ed) Total hip arthroplasty, vol II. Mosby, St. Louis, p 977
5. Hartofilakidis G, Karachalios T (2000) Total hip replacement in congenital hip disease. Surg Tech Orthop Traumatol 55:440-E-410
6. Hartofilakidis G, Karachalios T (2004) Total hip arthroplasty for congenital hip disease. J Bone Joint Surg Am 86-A(2):242–250
7. Brittain HA (1952) Architectural principles in arthrodesis, 2nd edn. E&S Livingstone, Edinburgh

Total hip replacement (THR) in patients with congenital hip disease (CHD), especially in cases with low and high dislocation, is difficult and may hide unexpected complications. The major technical difficulties, encountered during surgery, are reconstruction of the deficient acetabulum and implantation of the femoral component in cases with deformed upper femur and narrow and stovepipe-shaped diaphysis. Difficulties are even more increased in cases with angular deformities of the femur from previous osteotomies [1] (Fig. 3.4).

Basic principles for a successful uncomplicated THR in patients with CHD are:
- A wide exposure
- The restoration of the normal centre of rotation
- The use of special techniques and implants

7.1 Wide Exposure

A wide exposure is essential and is better achieved by the lateral transtrochanteric approach (TTA) (Fig. 7.1). The TTA was introduced by Charnley [2], who suggested that it would not only facilitate access to the joint but might also restore normal biomechanics by advancing the greater trochanter distally and laterally, thereby creating a more powerful abductor mechanism, by increasing the abductor lever arm, and minimises the reaction forces acting on the acetabulum [3, 4].

Charnley initially recommended the TTA for all THRs [2]. He believed that the problems arising from restricted exposure during surgery might lead to complications more serious than those occurring from the osteotomy itself (Fig. 7.2). He insisted that all orthopaedic surgeons should learn this approach, which would be needed in difficult hips and for revision operations. Although the majority of surgeons today prefer to use other approaches in routine primary cases, this method remains safe and effective in certain instances, including CHD, revision surgery, stiff hips, protrusio acetabuli and cases with severe osteoporosis [4].

Reattachment of the osteotomised greater trochanter is not always easy. This is due to shortened abductors, an often small and malpositioned trochanter and a lengthened limb. Four categories of the position of reattachment of the trochanter in relation to its original bed were recognised (Fig. 7.3): (a) reattachment at the original bed of trochanteric osteotomy; (b) distal reattachment in relation to its original bed, the trochanter having contact with the distal part of the original bed; (c) reattachment on the lateral femoral cortex in cases where the femoral neck was resected to the level of the distal part of the lesser trochanter and (d) reattachment proximal to its original bed [5].

Trochanteric non-union has remained a problem, with reported rates of up to 17 % in routine arthroplasties [6]. However, in a series of 192 THRs, presented by the authors exclusively in

Fig. 7.1 For a wide exposure, an extended incision and trochanteric osteotomy are necessary

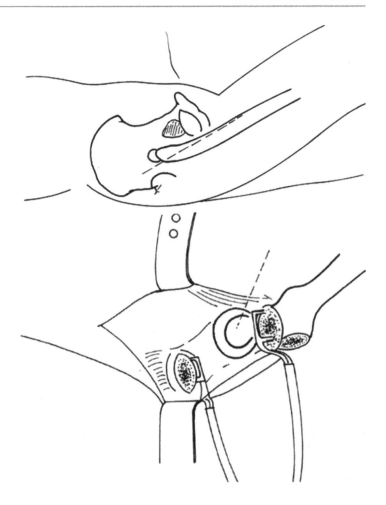

patients with CHD, the rate of non-union was 3 % (Fig. 7.4) [5]. As it is noted by Eftekhar, those surgeons performing trochanteric osteotomy routinely obtained a better rate of union than those reserving the procedure for cases with difficult anatomical problems [4]. The distinct advantages offered by the TTA in THR for patients with CHD far overweight the risk of non-union and other complications.

7.2 Restoration of the Normal Centre of Rotation

The anatomical placement (true acetabulum) of the acetabular component is recommended mainly for biomechanical reasons [1, 7, 8]. On the basis of a mathematical model of the hip joint, Johnston et al. [9] suggested that the displacement of the centre of rotation of the cemented acetabular component medially, inferiorly and anteriorly reduces hip loads significantly. High placement of the component in the region of false acetabulum has also been proposed [10, 11]. The disadvantage of this technique is that with the acetabular component at this level, the lever arm for the body weight is much longer than that of the abductors and causes excessive loading of the hip (Fig. 7.5). Also, the shearing forces acting on the acetabular component at a higher level can lead to early loosening. In addition, in unilateral cases a high acetabular component does not correct leg-length and leaves the patient with a limb.

Fig. 7.2 The surgeon of this patient decided not to osteotomise the greater trochanter. The result was a postoperative palsy of both femoral and peroneal nerve and an early loosening of the components within 2 years

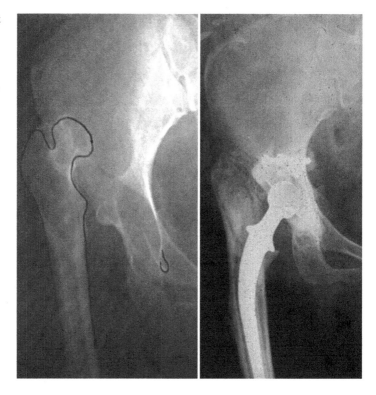

7.3   Reconstruction of the Acetabulum

In low dislocation, the true acetabulum has to be excavated underneath the inferior part of the false acetabulum by removing the osteophyte that covers the upper part of the true acetabulum. In high dislocation, the true acetabulum is identified by using the thickened and elongated joint capsule as guide. Once the true acetabulum is located, two Hohmann retractors are inserted as markers of the most distal and anterior boundaries of the true acetabulum. One retractor is inserted at the acetabular notch, which corresponds to the superior margin of the obturator foramen. The second retractor is inserted anteriorly, taking care to avoid the possibility of fracture, engaging the thin anterior wall, into the inner wall of the pelvis (Fig. 7.6) [12].

Once a wide exposure of the area of the true acetabulum has been achieved, the procedure follows the same steps in low and high dislocation. The hypoplastic true acetabulum is widened and deepened with small (38–40 mm) diameter reamers, directed superoposteriorly (Fig. 7.7). Deepening is continued until the outer surface of the internal pelvic cortex is reached. After preparation of the true acetabulum, a press fit small diameter cementless cup is inserted at an angle of 40–45° to the horizontal and with 10° anteversion, when the remaining osseous cavity can accommodate it with at least 70–80 % coverage of the implant with bone (Fig. 7.8). Due to the poor acetabular bone stock in most hips with CHD and to the effort during surgery to obtain stable fixation of the cementless acetabular component, it is not always possible by using these implants to obtain optimal inclination, positioning (vertical and horizontal distance to teardrop) and full osseous containment.

The inclination, horizontal and vertical placement, and bony containment of the cementless acetabular component inserted in patients with CHD has been reported that affect on the loosening of acetabular and femoral components, wear of polyethylene and periprosthetic osteolysis [13]. Concerning the positioning of the acetabular components, biomechanical analysis showed that

Fig. 7.3 Diagram showing the position of different sites of reattachment of the trochanter: (**a**) at its original bed; (**b**) distal reattachment, the trochanter retaining contact with the distal part of the original bed; (**c**) reattachment of the trochanter on the lateral femoral cortex; and (**d**) proximal reattachment

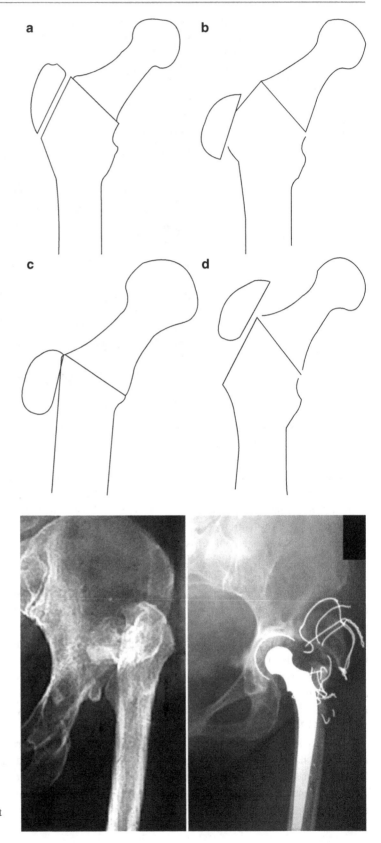

Fig. 7.4 Non-union of the trochanter in a case with high dislocation. As a result the patient remained with a Trendelenburg gait postoperatively

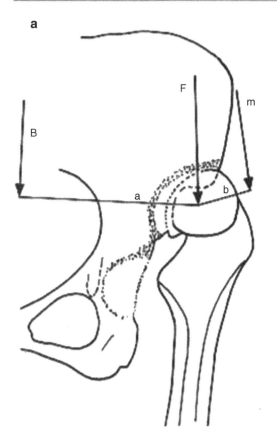

a

b

Fig. 7.5 (**a**) Forces acting on a hip with high dislocation: *B* body weight, *m* abductor force, *F* resultant force; *a* lever arm of the body weight, *b* lever arm of the abductors. (**b**) By restoring the normal centre of rotation of the hip, the lever arm of the abductors (*b*) becomes equal to the lever arm of the body weight (*a*) minimising loads acting on the hip

higher joint contact forces occurred with lateral placement of the cementless acetabular components in patients who did not have CHD [14].

If inclination, positioning and bony coverage at least 70–80 % of the cementless acetabular component cannot be achieved, the senior author (GH) suggests reconstruction of the acetabulum using the acetabuloplasty technique described and named cotyloplasty by K. Stamos (Fig. 7.9) [1, 3, 7, 15]

7.4 Classic Cotyloplasty Technique

A controlled comminuted fracture of the entire paper-thin medial wall of the acetabulum is created using the Charnley deepening reamer or a Lexer chisel or both. The reamer is struck lightly with a hammer until the entire floor of the acetabulum fractures. Care must be taken not to perforate the internal layer of the periosteum. A blind anchorage hole is then made with a Charnley starting drill in the roof of the acetabulum. A large amount of autogenous cancellous morselised (cut into small pieces) graft, taken from the femoral head and neck, is placed between the fragments of the acetabular floor and onto the periosteum of the fractured medial wall. The graft and the fragments of the acetabular floor are moulded and pushed slightly inwards with a hemispherical pusher or wrapped gauze or both.

A small size all-polyethylene acetabular component, usually the offset-bore cup, fully covered [16], is then cemented at an angle of 40–45° to the horizontal and with 10–15° anteversion, with minimal pressure being applied to avoid excessive medialisation (Fig. 7.10). This method of

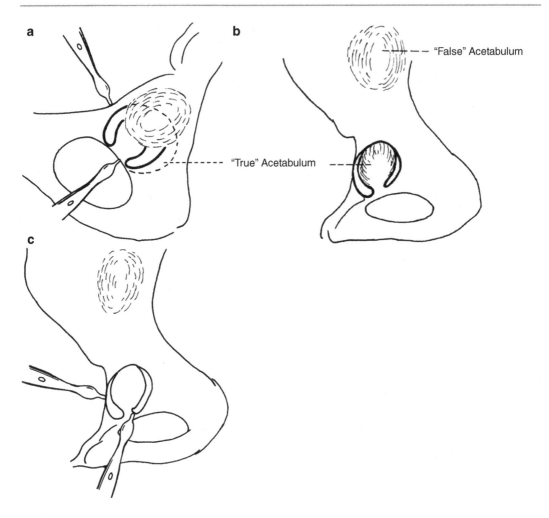

Fig. 7.6 (a) In low dislocation, the true acetabulum has to be excavated underneath the lower part of the false acetabulum. (b) In high dislocation, the true acetabulum is located following the elongated and thickened joint cap-

sule. (c) Two Hohmann retractors, one inserted at the acetabular notch and the other at the anterior wall, indicate the most distal and the anterior boundary of the true acetabulum

cotyloplasty creates abundant good-quality bone stock and allows medialisation of the acetabulum. Acrylic cement appears to bond satisfactorily to the bone grafts, as we have shown in experiments on dogs [17].

Dunn and Hess [18] proposed a similar technique, but with limited fragmentation of the medial wall, as well as reinforcement of the graft-cement interface with a wire mesh. A variety of different techniques, by advancing the medial wall of the acetabulum and by using morselised bone grafts, in combination with cementless components, has been described [19–24]. One of

the authors (GCB) is using for almost 10 years the Centroid Hilock cup that could be considered as a hybrid design that combines the benefits of the cementless fixation and the advantages of a ring fixed proximally to the roof of the acetabulum and distally with a hook in the obturator foramen in order to avoid protrusion. The use of a bulk structural autogenous graft from the femoral head to augment the superolateral aspect of the acetabular rim was proposed initially by Harris [10] with excellent short-term clinical results. However, a high rate of failure reported after approximately 12 years [25, 26] raised

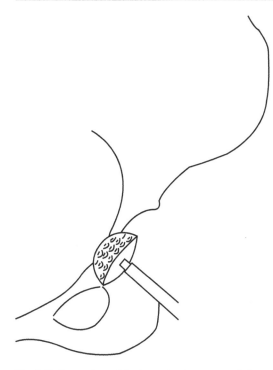

Fig. 7.7 Deepening of the hypoplastic true acetabulum, in low and high dislocations, is initiated with small diameter reamers (38–40 mm)

doubts as to the efficacy of this technique, and those who still recommend it rely considerably less on the bulk graft than on the host bone for support of the acetabular component (Fig. 7.11). The reason for such a high failure rate in this technique may be the complex pathological anatomy that we have described and the abnormal distribution of stresses combined with the unfavourable long-term biological behaviour of structural grafts (revascularisation, absorption and remodelling of the graft) [27].

7.5   Reconstruction of the Femur

In dysplastic hips and in the majority of hips with low dislocation, the reconstruction of the femur is similar to that of conventional cases. Problems arise with the more hypoplastic types of low dislocation and in hips with high dislocation. The narrow canal is prepared with hand-operated reamers, since power reamers may cause fracture or penetration of the thin cortex (Fig. 7.12). A trial reduction of the com-

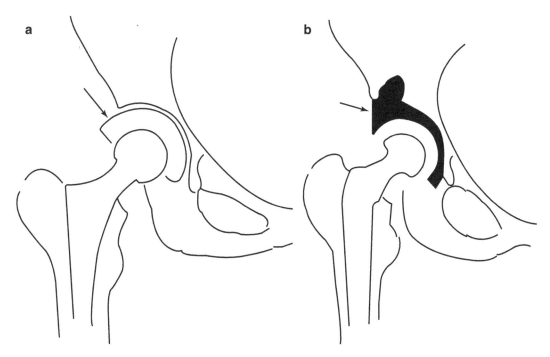

Fig. 7.8 For the reconstruction of the acetabulum, (**a**) cementless component can be used, when osseous cavity can accommodate it with at least 70–80 % coverage of the implant with host bone. (**b**) When cemented component is used, full coverage of the implant is necessary. *Arrows* indicate the extend of coverage of the acetabulum by host bone

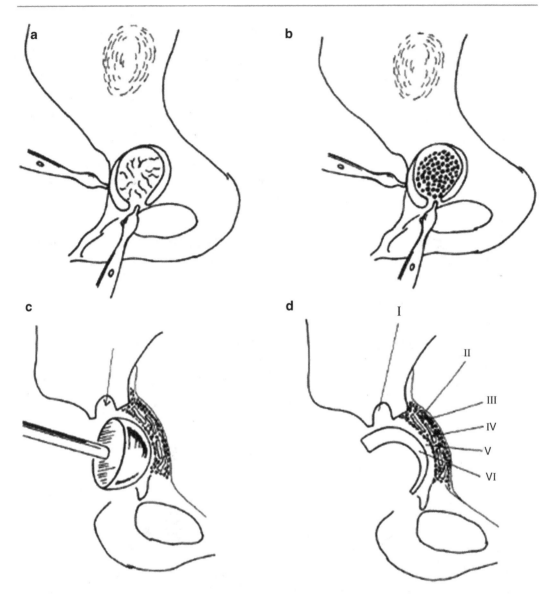

Fig. 7.9 Cotyloplasty technique: (**a**) comminuted fracture of the entire medial wall. (**b**) Large amount of cancellous morselised graft placed between the fragments of the acetabular floor, onto the periosteum. (**c**) Grafts moulded with a hemispherical pusher. (**d**) Final appearance: *I* anchorage hole, *II* internal layer of the periosteum, *III* autogenous morselised graft, *IV* fragments of the acetabular floor, *V* cement mantle, *VI* offset-bore acetabular component

ponents chosen, with the femoral component inserted at the correct degree of anteversion (approximately 10–15°), is attempted after release of the psoas tendon and the small external rotators. If the reduction is not possible, additional shortening of the femur is performed with progressive resection of the femoral neck (Fig. 7.13). Care is taken to keep the resection proximal to the lower part of the lesser trochanter; otherwise, the narrow diameter of the femoral canal, more distally, becomes a major problem. Shortening at the level of the neck of

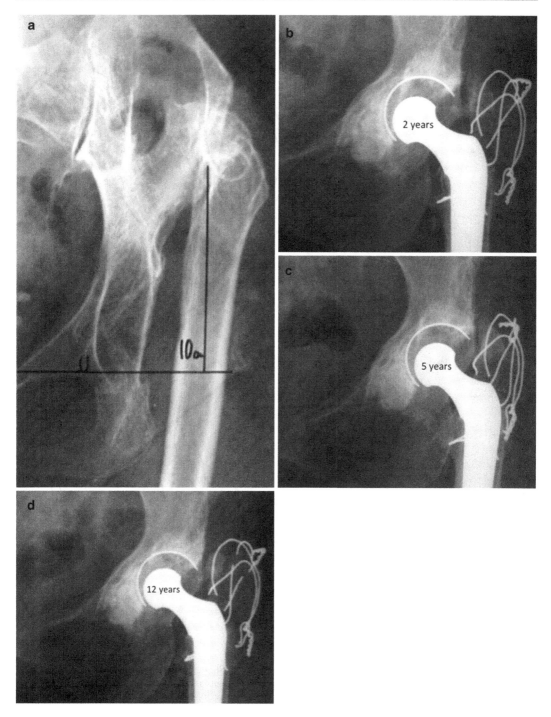

Fig. 7.10 (**a**) Radiograph of a 57-year-old female with high dislocation. Reconstruction of the acetabulum was performed by using the cotyloplasty technique and the offset-bore cup. Five months after surgery the incorporation of the grafts was completed. (**b**–**d**) Incorporation and viability of the grafts 2, 5 and 12 years postoperatively

Fig. 7.11 Drawings of (**a**) the use of bulk structural autogenous graft to augment the superolateral aspect of the acetabulum (Harris technique) and (**b**) the cotyloplasty technique (Stamos technique)

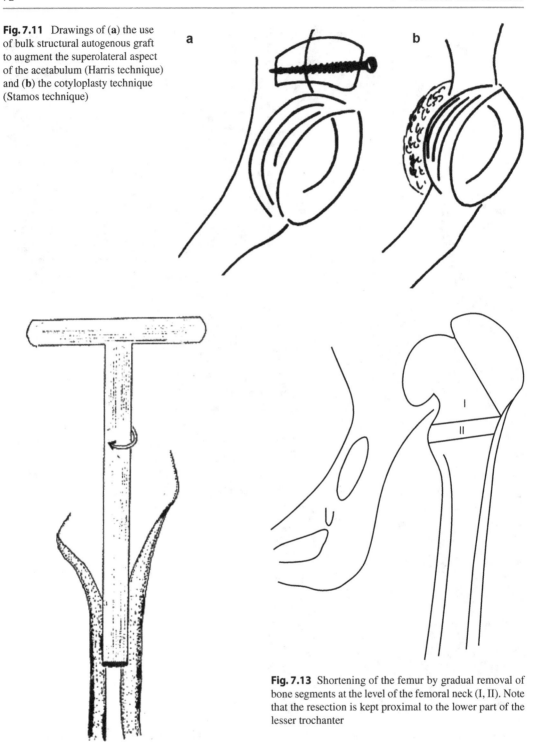

Fig. 7.13 Shortening of the femur by gradual removal of bone segments at the level of the femoral neck (I, II). Note that the resection is kept proximal to the lower part of the lesser trochanter

Fig. 7.12 Hand-operated reamer is used to prepare the narrow femoral canal

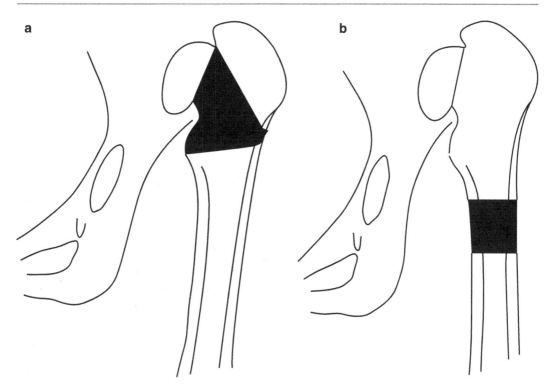

Fig. 7.14 Drawings of the two alternatives of shortening of the femur: (**a**) at the level of femoral neck and (**b**) distal shortening at the level of femoral shaft

the femur is simple and uneventful, and thus we do not favour subtrochanteric or distal shortening of the femoral diaphysis, as suggested by others (Fig. 7.14) [11, 28–31]. The creation of an artificial intraoperative fracture of the femur may itself cause undesirable complications. The prosthesis is then inserted, using so-called modern cementing techniques. The surgeon must be prepared to use a straight, thin prosthesis leaving adequate space for a cement mantle of sufficient width (Fig. 7.15). Special care must be taken to avoid inserting the stem with excess anteversion or in a varus or valgus position. In agreement with other authors, the senior author favours to use of cemented femoral prostheses. It is considered that the principles and goals of cementless fixation of the stems (optimal canal fit and fill, initial implant stability and adequate bone ingrowth) are not easily achievable in narrow femoral canals with such a thin cortex.

Currently new cementless designs are used. The new, thin, short Wagner-type designs, made of titanium with flutes with short neck, confer an easier, reproducible and safe method with mid-term good results for the femoral side [32]. One of the authors (GCB) is using these stems for approximately a decade.

Postoperatively, 2–3 weeks bed rest is recommended, with an abduction pillow between the legs for better adjustment and balance of the soft tissues. In cases of excessive lengthening, both the hip and the knee joint should be kept in moderate flexion for a few days with leg put on pillows to relieve tension on the femoral nerve (hip flexion) and on the sciatic nerve (knee flexion). The patient is instructed to start non-weight bearing walking the third postoperative week, while full weight bearing is usually permitted 3–4 months postoperatively. Other surgeons, using different techniques and implants, mobilise their patients much sooner with minimal weight bearing. Patients are advised to avoid passive adduction or active abduction to protect osteosynthesis of the greater trochanter for 6 weeks.

All patients enter in a THR registry and are examined at 3 and 6 weeks postoperatively and

Fig. 7.15 Two types of femoral stems most often used by the authors: (**a**) the Charnley CDH stem and (**b**) the Harris CDH stem

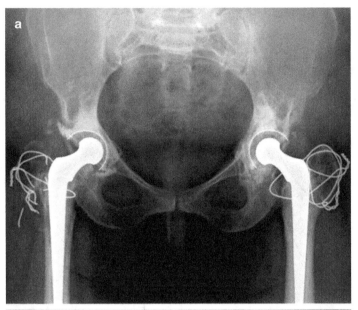

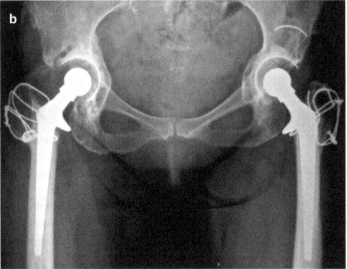

once every 1 or 2 years thereafter. Revision is undesirable, however can be successful if it is performed on time, before extensive bone destruction occurs.

References

1. Hartofilakidis G, Stamos K, Karachalios T (1998) Treatment of high dislocation of the hip in adults with total hip arthroplasty. Operative technique and long-term clinical results. J Bone Joint Surg Am 80(4): 510–517

2. Charnley J (1979) Low friction arthroplasty of the hip: theory and practice. Springer, Berlin

3. Hartofilakidis G, Stamos K, Ioannidis TT (1988) Low friction arthroplasty for old untreated congenital dislocation of the hip. J Bone Joint Surg Br 70(2):182–186

4. Eftekhar NS (1993) Congenital dysplasia and dislocation. In: Eftekhar NS (ed) Total hip arthroplasty, vol 2. Mosby, St. Louis, pp 905–908

5. Hartofilakidis G, Babis GC, Georgiades G, Kourlaba G (2011) Trochanteric osteotomy in total hip replacement for congenital hip disease. J Bone Joint Surg Br 93(5):601–607

6. Amstutz HC, Yao J (1991) Trochanteric non-union. In: Amstutz HC (ed) Hip arthroplasty. Churchill Livingstone, New York, p 457

7. Hartofilakidis G, Stamos K, Karachalios T, Ioannidis TT, Zacharakis N (1996) Congenital hip disease in adults. Classification of acetabular deficiencies and operative treatment with acetabuloplasty combined with total hip arthroplasty. J Bone Joint Surg Am 78(5):683–692

8. Karachalios T, Hartofilakidis G, Zacharakis N, Tsekoura M (1993) A 12- to 18-year radiographic follow-up study of Charnley low-friction arthroplasty. The role of the center of rotation. Clin Orthop Relat Res 296:140–147

9. Johnston RC, Brand RA, Crowninshield RD (1979) Reconstruction of the hip. A mathematical approach to determine optimum geometric relationships. J Bone Joint Surg Am 61(5):639–652

10. Harris WH, Crothers O, Oh I (1977) Total hip replacement and femoral-head bone-grafting for severe acetabular deficiency in adults. J Bone Joint Surg Am 59(6):752–759

11. Paavilainen T, Hoikka V, Paavolainen P (1993) Cementless total hip arthroplasty for congenitally dislocated or dysplastic hips. Technique for replacement with a straight femoral component. Clin Orthop Relat Res 297:71–81

12. Eftekar NS (1978) Variations in technique and specific considerations. In: Eftekar NS (ed) Principles of total hip arthroplasty. CV Mosby, St. Louis, pp 1–440

13. Georgiades G, Babis GC, Kourlaba G, Hartofilakidis G (2010) Effect of cementless acetabular component orientation, position, and containment in total hip arthroplasty for congenital hip disease. J Arthroplasty 25(7):1143–1150

14. Devane PA, Bourne RB, Rorabeck CH, Hardie RM, Horne JG (1995) Measurement of polyethylene wear in metal-backed acetabular cups. I. Three-dimensional technique. Clin Orthop Relat Res 319:303–316

15. Karachalios T, Roidis N, Lampropoulou-Adamidou K, Hartofilakidis G (2013) Acetabular reconstruction in patients with low and high dislocation: 20- to 32-year survival of an impaction grafting technique (named cotyloplasty). Bone Joint J 95-B(7): 887–892

16. Ioannidis TT, Zacharakis N, Magnissalis EA, Eliades G, Hartofilakidis G (1998) Long-term behaviour of the Charnley offset-bore acetabular cup. J Bone Joint Surg Br 80(1):48–53

17. Stamos KG, Karachalios T, Papagelopoulos PJ, Xenakis T, Korres DS, Koroneos E, Hartofilakidis G (2000) Long-term mechanical stability of the impacted morselized graft-cement interface in total joint replacement: an experimental study in dogs. Orthopedics 23(8):809–814

18. Dunn HK, Hess WE (1976) Total hip reconstruction in chronically dislocated hips. J Bone Joint Surg Am 58(6):838–845

19. Xenakis T, Koukoubis T, Hantes K, Varytimidis S, Soucacos PN (1997) Bone grafting in total hip arthroplasty for insufficient acetabulum. Acta Orthop Scand Suppl 275:33–37

20. Sanchez-Sotelo J, Berry DJ, Trousdale RT, Cabanela ME (2002) Surgical treatment of developmental dysplasia of the hip in adults: II. Arthroplasty options. J Am Acad Orthop Surg 10(5):334–344

21. Anderson MJ, Harris WH (1999) Total hip arthroplasty with insertion of the acetabular component without cement in hips with total congenital dislocation or marked congenital dysplasia. J Bone Joint Surg Am 81(3):347–354

22. Somford MP, Bolder SB, Gardeniers JW, Slooff TJ, Schreurs BW (2008) Favorable survival of acetabular reconstruction with bone impaction grafting in dysplastic hips. Clin Orthop Relat Res 466(2):359–365

23. Zhang H, Huang Y, Zhou YX, Lv M, Jiang ZH (2005) Acetabular medial wall displacement osteotomy in total hip arthroplasty: a technique to optimize the acetabular reconstruction in acetabular dysplasia. J Arthroplasty 20(5):562–567

24. Dorr LD, Tawakkol S, Moorthy M, Long W, Wan Z (1999) Medial protrusio technique for placement of a porous-coated, hemispherical acetabular component without cement in a total hip arthroplasty in patients who have acetabular dysplasia. J Bone Joint Surg Am 81(1):83–92

25. Harris WH (1993) Management of the deficient acetabulum using cementless fixation without bone grafting. Orthop Clin North Am 24(4):663–665

26. Mulroy RD Jr, Harris WH (1990) Failure of acetabular autogenous grafts in total hip arthroplasty. Increasing incidence: a follow-up note. J Bone Joint Surg Am 72(10):1536–1540

27. Goldberg VM, Stevenson S (1993) The biology of bone grafts. Semin Arthroplasty 4(2):58–63

28. Paavilainen T, Hoikka V, Solonen KA (1990) Cementless total replacement for severely dysplastic or dislocated hips. J Bone Joint Surg Br 72(2): 205–211

29. Pagnano WM, Hansen DA, Shaughnessy WF (1996) Developmental hip dysplasia. In: Morrey BF (ed) Reconstructive surgery of the joints. Churchill Livingstone, New York, pp 1013–1026

30. Papagelopoulos PJ, Trousdale RT, Lewallen DG (1996) Total hip arthroplasty with femoral osteotomy for proximal femoral deformity. Clin Orthop Relat Res 332:151–162

31. Symeonides PP, Pournaras J, Petsatodes G, Christoforides J, Hatzokos I, Pantazis E (1997) Total hip arthroplasty in neglected congenital dislocation of the hip. Clin Orthop Relat Res 341:55–61

32. Faldini C, Miscione MT, Chehrassan M, Acri F, Pungetti C, d'Amato M, Luciani D, Giannini S (2011) Congenital hip dysplasia treated by total hip arthroplasty using cementless tapered stem in patients younger than 50 years old: results after 12-years follow-up. J Orthop Traumatol 12(4):213–218

Complications and Results

8.1 Complications

It has been reported that complications associated with total hip replacement (THR) in patients with congenital hip disease (CHD) are higher, according to the severity of the disease, when compared to those in patients with primary osteoarthritis [1]. These complications include nerve palsies and dislocations.

Sciatic and femoral nerves are the most vulnerable nerves to be damaged during THR [2, 3]. The overall incidence of nerve palsy after THR has been reported to be 0.8–3.7 % [4], while in a large number of patients with CHD, Schmalzried et al. found prevalence of nerve palsies 5.2 % after THR [5]. Several authors have associated nerve palsies with leg-lengthening in cases with CHD. Farrell et al. [6] reported that the preoperative diagnosis of CHD and the leg-lengthening were associated significantly with the development of postoperative nerve palsies ($p=0.0004$ and $p<0.01$, respectively). There is a controversy regarding the safe amount of leg-lengthening among different authors. Garvin et al. considered the 2 cm [7], while Edwards et al. the 4 cm [8]. However, in 13 cases of our series where leg-lengthening surpassed 5 cm (5–7), no neurological complications were observed [9]. Also, Eggli et al. [10], in a series of 508 THRs for CHD, found no statistical correlation between the amount of leg-lengthening and the incidence of nerve damage ($p=0.47$), while they found significant correlation between nerve palsy and intraoperative difficulty ($p=0.041$) such as previous surgery, severe deformity, a defect of the acetabular roof or considerable flexion deformity.

Higher rates of postoperative dislocation, in patients with CHD, are also reported. The Norwegian Arthroplasty Registry [11] found that THRs for CHD have 5.6 times higher risk of revision due to dislocation when compared with THRs for primary osteoarthritis. The risk of postoperative dislocation has been reported to increase with trochanteric non-union, high hip centre, medialisation of the cup [12], small femoral head size [13, 14] and large acetabular component outer diameter [14].

Hypoplastic or deformed femoral diaphysis in hips with CHD leads to increased risk of intraoperative femoral fracture which is reported to range from 5 to 22 % [15], and therefore care must be taken when preparing the femoral canal to avoid cortical perforation (see Chap. 7). The postoperative infection rate is reported as higher as ten times in patients with CHD when compared to other diagnoses. This could be due to the complexity and duration of these operations, the large exposure and extensive dissection, soft tissue stripping and the frequent use of bone grafts [16].

We have registered the complications of 223 THRs performed in 162 patients with osteoarthritis secondary to CHD: 76 dysplastic hips, 69 hips with low dislocation and 84 hips with high dislocation [17]. In the dysplastic group, there was one postoperative femoral nerve palsy that resolved within 1 year. One patient with a low dislocation presented with palsy of both the

G. Hartofilakidis et al., *Congenital Hip Disease in Adults*,
DOI 10.1007/978-88-470-5492-9_8, © Springer-Verlag Italia 2014

peroneal and the femoral nerve on the fifteenth postoperative day, possibly as a result of a peri-neural hematoma. The femoral nerve palsy resolved completely within 6 months, but the peroneal nerve palsy resulted in a permanent incomplete drop foot. In the group of hips with a high dislocation, there was one peroneal nerve and one femoral nerve palsy. Both fully resolved within 6 months. Postoperative dislocations occurred in eight hips. In three hips, the acetabular component was revised because of incorrect orientation. Five dislocations occurred at 7–52 days following hybrid total hip arthroplasties (during the initial period of application of this method); one occurred in a hip with a low dislocation and four in hips with a high dislocation. Four of these dislocations were treated with closed reduction and one with open reduction. No recurrence of any of the eight dislocations was recorded. Femoral fracture occurred in a hip with low dislocation 22 years postoperatively and treated with internal fixation. One dysplastic hip, three hips with low dislocation and three with high dislocation developed deep infection.

To evaluate the complications associated with trochanteric osteotomy, we studied 192 THRs in 140 patients with CHD: 34 dysplastic hips, 93 with low dislocation and 65 with high dislocation [18]. The non-union rate of the osteotomy was 3 % (5 hips). Fibrous union was noticed in 29 hips (15 %) resulting in a mild Trendelenburg gait postoperatively. The rate of union had a statistically significant relationship with the position of reattachment of the trochanter, which depended greatly on the preoperative diagnosis. Acetabular and femoral loosening had a statistically significant relationship with defective union (non-union and fibrous union) and the position of reattachment of the trochanter. Different authors have reported that trochanteric osteotomy increases the risk of heterotopic ossification [19–22]. However, Brooker et al. [23] stated that unless there was ankylosis (Brooker IV), the functional result is not affected. In our series, Brooker grade IV heterotopic ossification was seen in only three hips (2 %) resulting in complete ankylosis in one hip (Fig. 8.1) and gross limitation of movement in the other two. We suggest that in routine cases of THR, trochanteric osteotomy may be optional,

but it remains a useful technique in cases with CHD, especially those with low and high dislocation.

With proper surgical technique and postoperative care, complications, especially nerve damage and postoperative dislocation, can be minimised. Nerve damage can be avoided by cautious handling of the various retractors intraoperatively and, in high or low dislocations, by the placement of both the hip and the knee in flexion for 3–4 days after the operation. Postoperative dislocation can be minimised by proper orientation of the cup (inclination of 30–45° in the frontal plane and 10–15° of anteversion).

8.2 Results

While reporting results of total hip replacement (THR), long-term follow-up is of paramount importance. Short-term results are unreliable.

The reported results of THR in patients with congenital hip disease (CHD) are not easily comparable (Table 8.1) [2, 7, 17, 24–40]. The material in the majority of reports is not homogenous, since they include different types of the disease, duration of follow-up, implants and techniques used and statistical analysis. In five relatively homogenous series of high dislocated hips that we are aware, it is reported 25 % failure rate in a group of 87 hips at an average 10 years (5–16) of follow-up [26], 14.7 % in a smaller group of 34 hips at an average 9.4 years (5.6–14) of follow-up [27], 12.7 % in a group of 118 hips at an average 12.8 years (10–26) of follow-up [33], 17 % in a group of 116 hips at an average 9.7 years (6–14) of follow-up [36] and 20 % in a group of 20 hips at an average 10.2 years (5–20) of follow-up [40].

In our experience, based on a cohort of 84 hips in 67 female patients with high dislocation who underwent THR during the years of 1976–1994, the survival rate was 92.4 % at 5 years, 88.0 % at 10 years, 76.4 % at 15 years and 53 % at 20 years [17, 39, 41]. It was noted that the 64 hips that underwent Charnley low-friction arthroplasty had an increased revision rate with time, equally due to loosening of the acetabular cup or the femoral stem. In the 19 hips with hybrid total hip

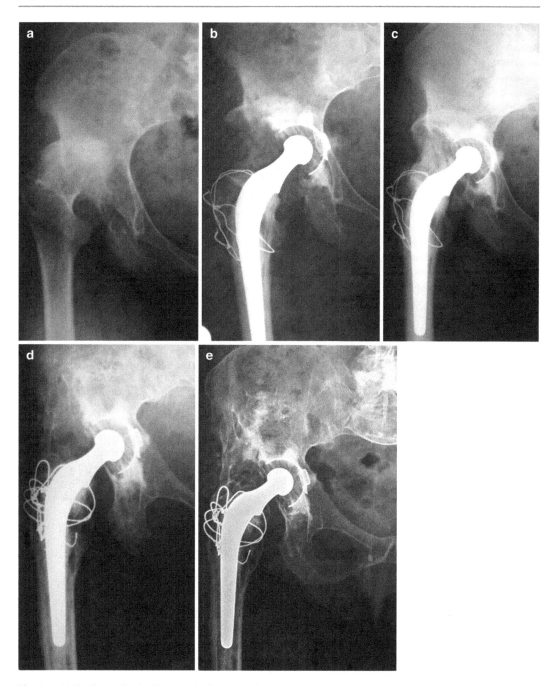

Fig. 8.1 (**a**) Radiograph of a 43-year-old female patient with low dislocation of B2 subtype on the right hip. (**b**) Two months after low-friction arthroplasty. (**c**) Radiograph 1 year after surgery with complete ankylosis due to Brooker IV heterotopic ossification. (**d**) Radiograph after excision of the largest part of the heterotopic ossification. Patient regained 70° of flexion, 15° abduction, 10° adduction and 15° of external rotation. (**e**) Final radiograph taken 34 years after primary surgery

replacement, the main reason for revision was progressive wear of the polyethylene acetabular liner [39]. Our relatively favourable clinical results and long-term survival of THR in patients with high dislocation indicate that a thorough understanding of anatomical abnormalities and the use of proper reconstruction techniques and implants make THR feasible in patients who

Table 8.1 Mid- and long-term reported results of THR

Year of publication	Authors	No of hips	Range of follow-up (years)	CHD type (no of hips)	Failure rate (%)
1979	Crowe et al. [2]	31	2–6	Severe dysplasia, dislocation	9.7
1988	Linde et al. [24]	129	Not referred	Congenital dislocation and subluxation	11
1991	Fredin et al. [25]	21	5–11	Crowe type IV	23.8
1991	Garvin et al. [7]	23	8–16.5	Severe dysplasia, dislocation	26.0
1991	Kavanaugh et al. [26]	87	5–16	Complete dislocation	25
1993	Anwar et al. [27]	34	5.6–14	Congenital dislocation	14.7
1993	Paavilainen et al. [28]	67	3–5	Severe dysplasia, dislocation	44.8
1995	Morscher [29]	71	1–9	Dysplasia, dislocation	12.7
1996	MacKenzie et al. [30]	59	10–21	Crowe type II, III, IV	13.6
1997	Nagano et al. [31]	34	15–23.3	Congenital hip dysplasia	11.8
1997	Numair et al. [32]	232	3.1–22.8	Crowe type I, II, III (136)	9[a]
					3[b]
				Type IV (46)	15[a]
					2[b]
2001	Kerboull et al. [33]	118	10–26	Crowe type IV	12.7
2003	Ito et al. [34]	81	8–15	Hartofilakidis type I (70), II (7), III (4)	2.5
2004	Hartofilakidis and Karachalios [17]	223	7–26	Hartofilakidis type I (76)	21
				Type II (69)	28
				Type III (84)	22
2005	Chougle et al. [35]	292	2.2–31.2	Hartofilakidis type I (215), II (55), III (22)	26.4
2005	Kim and Kim [36]	116	6–14	Hartofilakidis type I (40)	5
				Type II (34)	9
				Type III (42)	17
2005	Klapach et al. [37]	66	20–30	Crowe type II, III, IV	12
2009	Bruzzone et al. [38]	100	4–18	Developmental dysplasia of the hip	10[a]
					1[b]
2011	Hartofilakidis et al. [39]	84	15–33	Hartofilakidis type III	44
2012	Hasegawa et al. [40]	20	5–20	Crowe type IV	20

[a]For the acetabular component only
[b]For the femoral component only

have such complex CHD. These findings may be useful for comparison with the results of THR performed with newer surgical techniques and implant designs in a similar group of patients.

It is generally agreed that the clinical and radiographic results of THR, performed for degenerative arthritis secondary to CHD, vary depending on the severity of the anatomical abnormalities. The senior author (GH) reported on 223 consecutive primary THRs in 162 patients with osteoarthritis secondary to CHD [17]. Seventy-six hips were dysplastic, 69 had a low dislocation and 84 had a high dislocation (Figs. 8.2 and 8.3). The overall rate of failure for the dysplastic hips, the hips with a low dislocation and those with a high dislocation was 21, 28 and 22 % at 7–26 years of follow-up, with an overall 15-year survivorship 88.8, 73.9 and 76.4 %, respectively. Specifically, the rate of revision of the acetabular component was 15 %

Fig. 8.2 (**a**) Radiograph of a 52-year-old patient with low dislocation of both hips. (**b**) Radiograph 39 years after low-friction arthroplasty in both hips. Note that the cement mantle is not visible due to its radiolucency at that time

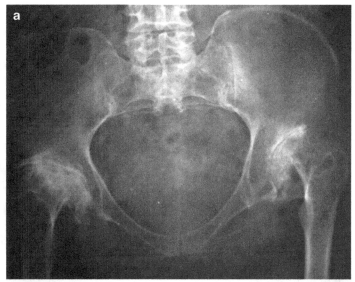

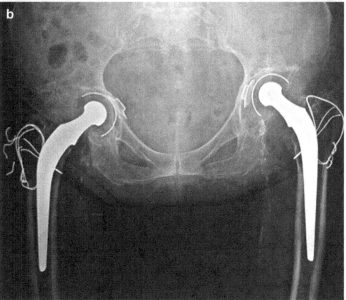

for the dysplastic hips, 21 % for the hips with a low dislocation and 14 % for the hips with a high dislocation, and of the femoral component it was 14, 14 and 16 %, respectively. When the revision rates of both the acetabular and the femoral components were compared among the three types of disease, no significant differences were found. In patients with a low dislocation, the major technical problem was reconstruction of the acetabulum, and in those with a high dislocation, the challenge was to place the acetabular component

inside the reconstructed true acetabulum and to use an appropriate femoral implant in the hypoplastic narrow femoral diaphysis.

8.2.1 Authors' Related Publications

- Acetabular reconstruction in patients with low and high dislocation. 20–32 years survival of an impaction grafting technique (named cotyloplasty) (2013) *Bone Joint J* [42]

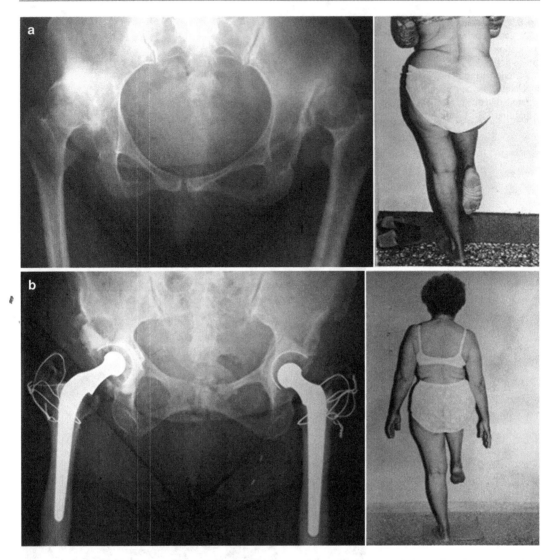

Fig. 8.3 (**a**) Radiograph of a 40-year-old female with high dislocation on the left hip and low on the right. The patient presents positive Trendelenburg sign. (**b**) Radiograph 33 and 28 years after low-friction arthroplasty on the right and left hip, respectively. After surgery, the Trendelenburg sign became negative

We reported the results of 61 THRs, carried out on 44 patients with low and high dislocation, performed after reconstruction of the acetabulum with the cotyloplasty technique (Figs. 11.25 and 11.26). The patients were followed postoperatively for 20–32 years. Twenty-eight (49 %) acetabular components were revised because of aseptic loosening at an average of 16 years (6–26) after the index operation. The overall survival rate was 93.1 % (±6.5 %) at 10 years and 56.1 % (±13.3 %) at 23 when 22 hips remained at risk.

These long-term results are considered satisfactory for the reconstruction of an acetabulum presenting inadequate bone stock and circumferential segmental defects, as in hips with low and high dislocation. These results may be used in comparisons of outcomes with different techniques used to reconstruct the deficiencies of the acetabulum during THR in this type of hips.

- Results of total hip arthroplasty differ in subtypes of high dislocation (2013) *Clin Orthop Relat Res* [43]

We investigated differences in the results of THR between subtypes of high dislocation of the hip depending on the presence (C1) or absence (C2) of a false acetabulum (Figs. 6.4, 11.16, 11.17 and 11.18). In this study were included 49 hips of C1 subtype and 30 of C2 subtype. The 15-year survival was 84 % (±10 %) for the C1 subtype and 60 % (±17 %) for the C2 subtype ($p = 0.001$) [43]. To our knowledge there are no other studies in the literature comparing the long-term results of THR in high dislocation subtypes. The differences in survivorships seem reasonable because C2-type hips have more affected morphology compared with C1-type hips that may result in a higher rate of failure [44, 45]. These findings indicate that when reporting results of THR in patients with high dislocation, mixing results of the two subtypes may lead to statistical bias. It is therefore important that these subtypes be stratified in analyses that deal with the survivorship of THRs.

• Long-term behaviour of the Charnley offset-bore acetabular cup (1998) *J Bone Joint Surg Br* [46]

The Charnley offset-bore socket is an extra small implant with a face diameter of 35 mm and an eccentric cavity for the femoral head. The thickness of the polyethylene is approximately 10 mm in the upper weight bearing part, equal to that of conventional sockets, and then decreases to a few millimetres in the lower part. We reported the midterm radiographic results, after a mean of 7 years (3–19) follow-up of 58 THRs, performed between 1976 and 1997, using the offset-bore socket. In 44 hips the offset-bore socket was used in combination with cotyloplasty. All patients were women with a mean age of 48.4. Five sockets were revised at a mean of 9.8 years (4–16). At the mean follow-up of 7 years, the wear rate was 0.06 and 0.04 mm/year, respectively, in zones I and II of DeLee and Charnley.

Updated results at a minimum of 18 years (18–34) of the same cohort of 58 offset-bore sockets showed that 25 more sockets were revised. Thus, in total 30 sockets (52 %) were revised at a mean of 15 years (4–28). One hip was infected postoperatively and converted to Girdlestone. Five patients (7 hips) died

14–19 years (mean 16 years) retaining the initial implant. Fifteen patients (20 hips) are living at a mean age of 81 (53–86) with the initial implant in situ for a mean of 23 years (20–34) [47] (Figs. 11.17 and 11.18).

To our knowledge, the offset-bore socket is not anymore available. Newer implants, cemented and cementless, that are used need to be further considered, in comparison with the results obtained with the use of the offset-bore cup.

• Evaluation of two surgical techniques for acetabular reconstruction in total hip replacement for congenital hip disease: results after a minimum 10-year follow-up (2008) *J Bone Joint Surg Br* [48]

We have evaluated the results of THR in patients with CHD using 46 cemented all-polyethylene Charnley acetabular components implanted with the cotyloplasty technique in 34 patients (group A) and compared them with 47 metal-backed cementless acetabular components implanted without bone grafting in 33 patients (group B). Patients in group A were treated between 1988 and 1993 and those in group B between 1990 and 1995. The mean follow-up for group A was 16.6 years (12–18) and the mean follow-up for group B was 13.4 years (10–16). Revision for aseptic loosening was undertaken in 15 hips (32.6 %) in group A and in four hips (8.5 %) in group B. When liner exchange was included, a total of 13 hips was revised in group B (27.7 %). The mean polyethylene wear was 0.11 mm/year (0.002–0.43) and 0.107 mm/year (0–0.62) for groups A and B, respectively. Polyethylene wear in group A was associated with linear osteolysis and in group B with expansile osteolysis. In the event of failure of the liner in the presence of a well-fixed metal shell, it is possible to undertake early intervention with exchange of the worn liner prior to the development of extensive osteolysis. The introduction of improved designs with a more stable locking mechanism, the use of the cross-linked polyethylene and the potential to use hard-on-hard bearings may lead to longer survival of the cementless components used for reconstruction of the acetabulum. Cotyloplasty remains a reliable alternative in selected cases.

- Effect of cementless acetabular component orientation, position, and containment in total hip arthroplasty for congenital hip disease (2010) J Arthroplasty [49]

We evaluated the effect of the inclination angle, position and containment of 53 cementless cups inserted in patients with CHD, after a minimum of 10 years of follow-up. The polyethylene wear rate was significantly greater when the cup was placed in more than 45° inclination ($p = 0.045$) or if the cup was placed lateral to the teardrop position by more than 25 mm ($p = 0.001$). Aseptic loosening of the femoral component was significantly greater when the cup was placed more than 25 mm superiorly to the teardrop ($p = 0.049$). Cup placement of more than 25 mm lateral to the teardrop affected significantly peri-acetabular osteolysis ($p = 0.032$). The current study underlines the importance of optimising the angle of inclination, the position and the bony containment of the cementless metal-backed acetabular components during THR for CHD. If a choice must be made, it is preferable to avoid vertical inclination and lateral and superior placements of the cup in an attempted to obtain better bony coverage given that the cup is stable even with 70–80 % containment. If this is not possible, other surgical techniques should be considered.

- The twenty-year survivorship of two CDH stems with different design features (2012) *Eur J Orthop Surg Traumatol* [50]

Previous studies have shown that anatomical abnormalities of the femur in dislocated hips require the application of special CDH prosthesis for the reconstruction of the proximal femur in THR. We have retrospectively examined the clinical records and radiographs of 50 patients (67 hips) with low and high dislocations treated with THR in our institution, between 1987 and 1994. For the reconstruction of the femur, the stainless steel Charnley CDH stem, with polished surface, monoblock and collarless, was used in 32 hips; the Harris CDH stem, made of CoCr, precoated at the proximal part, modular and with collar, was used in 35 hips (see Fig. 7.15). At the time of the latest follow-up, 11 Charnley and 6 Harris CDH stems had been revised for aseptic loosening at an average of 14 years (6–20) and 13 years

(2–19), respectively. The survival rate at 20 years, with failure for aseptic loosening as the end point, was 63 % for the Charnley and 78 % for the Harris CDH stems. These results provide a basis for evaluation of newer techniques and designs.

References

1. Cameron HU, Botsford DJ, Park YS (1996) Influence of the Crowe rating on the outcome of total hip arthroplasty in congenital hip dysplasia. J Arthroplasty 11(5):582–587
2. Crowe JF, Mani VJ, Ranawat CS (1979) Total hip replacement in congenital dislocation and dysplasia of the hip. J Bone Joint Surg Am 61(1):15–23
3. Cameron HU, Eren OT, Solomon M (1998) Nerve injury in the prosthetic management of the dysplastic hip. Orthopedics 21(9):980–981
4. Oldenburg M, Muller RT (1997) The frequency, prognosis and significance of nerve injuries in total hip arthroplasty. Int Orthop 21(1):1–3
5. Schmalzried TP, Amstutz HC, Dorey FJ (1991) Nerve palsy associated with total hip replacement. Risk factors and prognosis. J Bone Joint Surg Am 73(7): 1074–1080
6. Farrell CM, Springer BD, Haidukewych GJ, Morrey BF (2005) Motor nerve palsy following primary total hip arthroplasty. J Bone Joint Surg Am 87(12): 2619–2625
7. Garvin KL, Bowen MK, Salvati EA, Ranawat CS (1991) Long-term results of total hip arthroplasty in congenital dislocation and dysplasia of the hip. A follow-up note. J Bone Joint Surg Am 73(9):1348–1354
8. Edwards BN, Tullos HS, Noble PC (1987) Contributory factors and etiology of sciatic nerve palsy in total hip arthroplasty. Clin Orthop Relat Res 218: 136–141
9. Hartofilakidis G, Karachalios T (2000) Total hip replacement in congenital hip disease. Surg Tech Orthop Traumatol 55:440-E-410
10. Eggli S, Hankemayer S, Muller ME (1999) Nerve palsy after leg lengthening in total replacement arthroplasty for developmental dysplasia of the hip. J Bone Joint Surg Br 81(5):843–845
11. Furnes O, Lie SA, Espehaug B, Vollset SE, Engesaeter LB, Havelin LI (2001) Hip disease and the prognosis of total hip replacements. A review of 53,698 primary total hip replacements reported to the Norwegian Arthroplasty Register 1987-99. J Bone Joint Surg Br 83(4):579–586
12. Malik A, Maheshwari A, Dorr LD (2007) Impingement with total hip replacement. J Bone Joint Surg Am 89(8):1832–1842
13. Wang L, Trousdale RT, Ai S, An KN, Dai K, Morrey BF (2012) Dislocation after total hip arthroplasty among patients with developmental dysplasia of the hip. J Arthroplasty 27(5):764–769

14. Kelley SS, Lachiewicz PF, Hickman JM, Paterno SM (1998) Relationship of femoral head and acetabular size to the prevalence of dislocation. Clin Orthop Relat Res 355:163–170

15. Reikeras O, Haaland JE, Lereim P (2010) Femoral shortening in total hip arthroplasty for high developmental dysplasia of the hip. Clin Orthop Relat Res 468(7):1949–1955

16. Sochart DH, Porter ML (1997) The long-term results of Charnley low-friction arthroplasty in young patients who have congenital dislocation, degenerative osteoarthrosis, or rheumatoid arthritis. J Bone Joint Surg Am 79(11):1599–1617

17. Hartofilakidis G, Karachalios T (2004) Total hip arthroplasty for congenital hip disease. J Bone Joint Surg Am 86-A(2):242–250

18. Hartofilakidis G, Babis GC, Georgiades G, Kourlaba G (2011) Trochanteric osteotomy in total hip replacement for congenital hip disease. J Bone Joint Surg Br 93(5):601–607

19. DeLee J, Ferrari A, Charnley J (1976) Ectopic bone formation following low friction arthroplasty of the hip. Clin Orthop Relat Res 121:53–59

20. Errico TJ, Fetto JF, Waugh TR (1984) Heterotopic ossification. Incidence and relation to trochanteric osteotomy in 100 total hip arthroplasties. Clin Orthop Relat Res 190:138–141

21. Morrey BF, Adams RA, Cabanela ME (1984) Comparison of heterotopic bone after anterolateral, transtrochanteric, and posterior approaches for total hip arthroplasty. Clin Orthop Relat Res 188: 160–167

22. Vicar AJ, Coleman CR (1984) A comparison of the anterolateral, transtrochanteric, and posterior surgical approaches in primary total hip arthroplasty. Clin Orthop Relat Res 188:152–159

23. Brooker AF, Bowerman JW, Robinson RA, Riley LH Jr (1973) Ectopic ossification following total hip replacement. Incidence and a method of classification. J Bone Joint Surg Am 55(8):1629–1632

24. Linde F, Jensen J, Pilgaard S (1988) Charnley arthroplasty in osteoarthritis secondary to congenital dislocation or subluxation of the hip. Clin Orthop Relat Res 227:164–171

25. Fredin H, Sanzen L, Sigurdsson B, Unander-Scharin L (1991) Total hip arthroplasty in high congenital dislocation. 21 hips with a minimum five-year follow-up. J Bone Joint Surg Br 73(3):430–433

26. Kavanaugh BF, Shaughnessy WJ, Fitzgerald RH (1991) Congenital dislocation of the hip. In: Morrey BF (ed) Joint replacement arthroplasty. Churchill Livingstone, London, pp 745–747

27. Anwar MM, Sugano N, Masuhara K, Kadowaki T, Takaoka K, Ono K (1993) Total hip arthroplasty in the neglected congenital dislocation of the hip. A five- to 14-year follow-up study. Clin Orthop Relat Res 295: 127–134

28. Paavilainen T, Hoikka V, Paavolainen P (1993) Cementless total hip arthroplasty for congenitally dislocated or dysplastic hips. Technique for replacement with a straight femoral component. Clin Orthop Relat Res 297:71–81

29. Morscher EW (1995) Total hip replacement for osteoarthritis in congenital hip dysplasia. Eur Instr Course Lect 2:1–8

30. MacKenzie JR, Kelley SS, Johnston RC (1996) Total hip replacement for coxarthrosis secondary to congenital dysplasia and dislocation of the hip. Long-term results. J Bone Joint Surg Am 78(1):55–61

31. Nagano H, Inoue H, Usui M, Mitani S, Satoh T (1997) Long-term results of Charnley low-friction arthroplasty for coxarthrosis with congenital hip dysplasia. 15 year follow-up study. Bull Hosp Jt Dis 56(4):197–203

32. Numair J, Joshi AB, Murphy JC, Porter ML, Hardinge K (1997) Total hip arthroplasty for congenital dysplasia or dislocation of the hip. Survivorship analysis and long-term results. J Bone Joint Surg Am 79(9): 1352–1360

33. Kerboull M, Hamadouche M, Kerboull L (2001) Total hip arthroplasty for Crowe type IV developmental hip dysplasia: a long-term follow-up study. J Arthroplasty 16(8 Suppl 1):170–176

34. Ito H, Matsuno T, Minami A, Aoki Y (2003) Intermediate-term results after hybrid total hip arthroplasty for the treatment of dysplastic hips. J Bone Joint Surg Am 85-A(9):1725–1732

35. Chougle A, Hemmady MV, Hodgkinson JP (2005) Severity of hip dysplasia and loosening of the socket in cemented total hip replacement. A long-term follow-up. J Bone Joint Surg Br 87(1):16–20

36. Kim YH, Kim JS (2005) Total hip arthroplasty in adult patients who had developmental dysplasia of the hip. J Arthroplasty 20(8):1029–1036

37. Klapach AS, Callaghan JJ, Miller KA, Goetz DD, Sullivan PM, Pedersen DR, Johnston RC (2005) Total hip arthroplasty with cement and without acetabular bone graft for severe hip dysplasia. A concise follow-up, at a minimum of twenty years, of a previous report. J Bone Joint Surg Am 87(2): 280–285

38. Bruzzone M, La Russa M, Garzaro G, Ferro A, Rossi P, Castoldi F, Rossi R (2009) Long-term results of cementless anatomic total hip replacement in dysplastic hips. Chir Organi Mov 93(3):131–136

39. Hartofilakidis G, Karachalios T, Georgiades G, Kourlaba G (2011) Total hip arthroplasty in patients with high dislocation: a concise follow-up, at a minimum of fifteen years, of previous reports. J Bone Joint Surg Am 93(17):1614–1618

40. Hasegawa Y, Iwase T, Kanoh T, Seki T, Matsuoka A (2012) Total hip arthroplasty for Crowe type developmental dysplasia. J Arthroplasty 27(9):1629–1635

41. Hartofilakidis G, Stamos K, Karachalios T (1998) Treatment of high dislocation of the hip in adults with total hip arthroplasty. Operative technique and long-term clinical results. J Bone Joint Surg Am 80(4): 510–517

42. Karachalios T, Roidis N, Lampropoulou-Adamidou K, Hartofilakidis G (2013) Acetabular reconstruction

in patients with low and high dislocation: 20- to 32-year survival of an impaction grafting technique (named cotyloplasty). Bone Joint J 95-B(7):887–892

43. Hartofilakidis G, Babis GC, Lampropoulou-Adamidou K, Vlamis J (2013) Results of total hip arthroplasty differ in subtypes of high dislocation. Clin Orthop Relat Res 471(9):2972–2979

44. Karachalios T, Hartofilakidis G (2010) Congenital hip disease in adults: terminology, classification, preoperative planning and management. J Bone Joint Surg Br 92(7):914–921

45. Xu H, Zhou Y, Liu Q, Tang Q, Yin J (2010) Femoral morphologic differences in subtypes of high developmental dislocation of the hip. Clin Orthop Relat Res 468(12):3371–3376

46. Ioannidis TT, Zacharakis N, Magnissalis EA, Eliades G, Hartofilakidis G (1998) Long-term behaviour of the Charnley offset-bore acetabular cup. J Bone Joint Surg Br 80(1):48–53

47. Hartofilakidis G (2010) Long-term behaviour of the Charnley offset-bore acetabular cup. unpublished data

48. Hartofilakidis G, Georgiades G, Babis GC, Yiannakopoulos CK (2008) Evaluation of two surgical techniques for acetabular reconstruction in total hip replacement for congenital hip disease: results after a minimum ten-year follow-up. J Bone Joint Surg Br 90(6):724–730

49. Georgiades G, Babis GC, Kourlaba G, Hartofilakidis G (2010) Effect of cementless acetabular component orientation, position, and containment in total hip arthroplasty for congenital hip disease. J Arthroplasty 25(7):1143–1150

50. Digas G, Georgiades G, Lampropoulou-Adamidou K, Hartofilakidis G (2012) The twenty-year survivorship of two CDH stems with different design features. Eur J Orthop Surg Traumatol [Epub ahead of print]

Difficult Cases

Total hip replacement (THR) in low and high dislocation is a difficult operation because of the anatomical features of these hips. Previous unsuccessful treatments increase considerably the surgical difficulties. Regardless the method and implants used for the reconstruction of these hips, wide exposure is mandatory and it is achieved when greater trochanter is osteotomised. Also, proximal shortening of the femur, when needed, facilitates the reconstruction of these difficult cases.

Clinical and radiological results in the majority of these cases are less satisfactory and reoperations more often. Examples are following (all patients were females).

Case 1

A 48-year-old patient with severe bilateral secondary osteoarthritis (OA) due to low dislocation. Both hips were stiff and almost fixed in 40° flexion. The patient at the age of 33 had in an other institution an intertrochanteric osteotomy on the left hip (Figs. 9.1, 9.2 and 9.3).

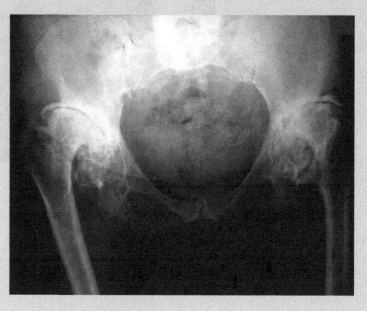

Fig. 9.1 Preoperative radiograph

G. Hartofilakidis et al., *Congenital Hip Disease in Adults*,
DOI 10.1007/978-88-470-5492-9_9, © Springer-Verlag Italia 2014

Fig. 9.2 One year after low-friction arthroplasty (LFA) of both hips. The patient gained compensatory range of motion and almost full level of activity

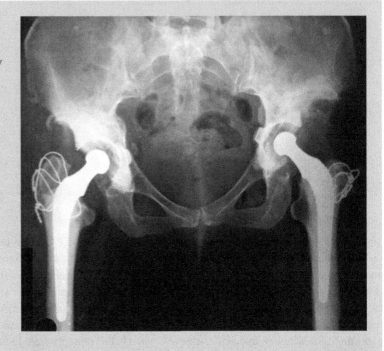

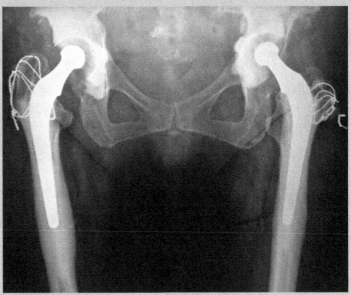

Fig. 9.3 Twenty years after surgery. The good result remains

Case 2

A 37-year-old patient with low dislocation of both hips. In 1952, at the age of 4, she had an operation of unknown type on the left hip followed by prolonged immobilisation in hip spica for 2.5 years according to patient's statement (Figs. 9.4, 9.5, 9.6 and 9.7).

Fig. 9.4 Preoperative radiographs. The left leg was 10 cm shorter probably due to the previous operation in childhood

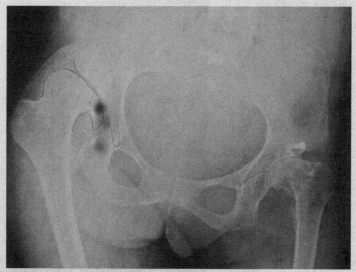

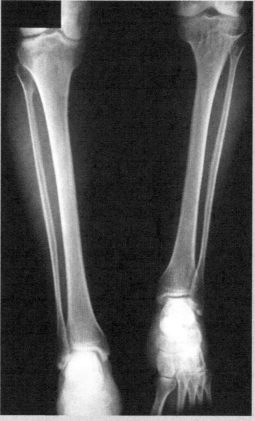

Fig. 9.5 Ten years after bilateral LFA. The cotyloplasty technique was used in both hips with offset-bore cups. In the femoral side, the CDH stems of Charnley were used. Seven centimetre shortening remained on the left leg

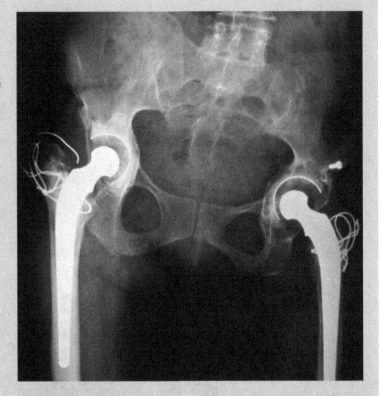

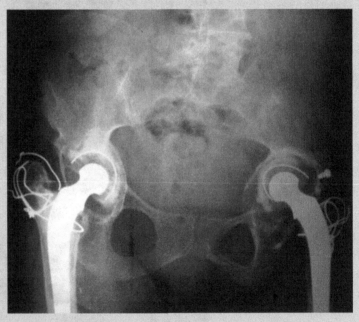

Fig. 9.6 Nineteen years postoperatively both acetabular components were loose and needed revision

Fig. 9.7 Seven years after revision of both components on both hips. Patient has no pain but a limited level of activity. For the acetabuli, cementless Hilock cups (Symbios) were used, and for the femoral side, cementless modular revision stems (Profemur, Wright)

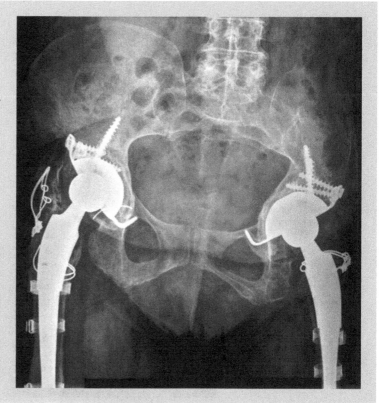

Case 3

Thirty-four-year-old patient with high dislocation on the right hip and dysplasia on the left. According to her medical record, at the age of 4 (1957), she had Schanz osteotomies on both hips (Figs. 9.8, 9.9 and 9.10).

Fig. 9.8 Preoperative radiograph. Reconstruction of both hips was performed as follows: (1) THR on the right hip by shortening of the femur at the level of the neck. (2) Corrective osteotomy of the left hip. (3) THR on the left hip (see also Fig. 6.7)

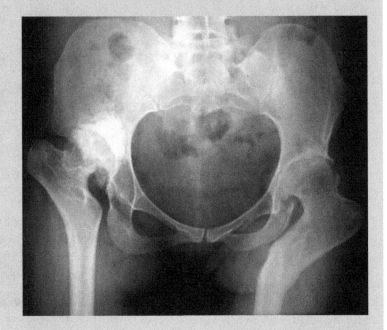

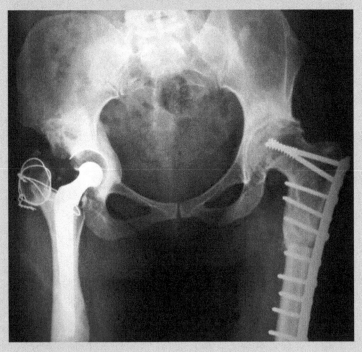

Fig. 9.9 Radiograph after LFA with cotyloplasty and offset-bore acetabular component on the right hip and corrective osteotomy on the left. After 2 years, a hybrid THR was followed on the left hip

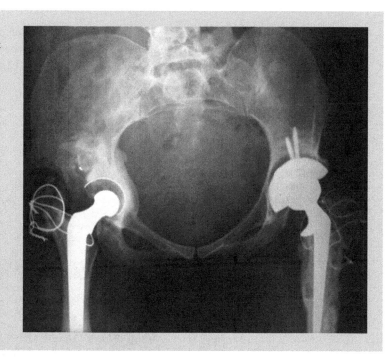

Fig. 9.10 Latest follow-up radiograph when the patient was 45 years old. She died 2 years later from breast cancer

Case 4

This patient with high dislocation of the left hip was examined by us when she was 62 years old. A Schanz osteotomy was performed in 1963 when she was 35 years old (Figs. 9.11 and 9.12).

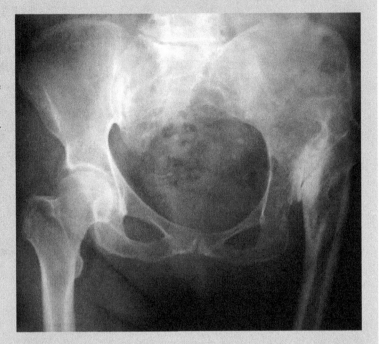

Fig. 9.11 Preoperative radiograph. The height of the dislocation was 9 cm. A cemented THR was followed using cotyloplasty technique and an offset-bore cup for the reconstruction of the acetabulum, and the Harris CDH stem for the reconstruction of the femur

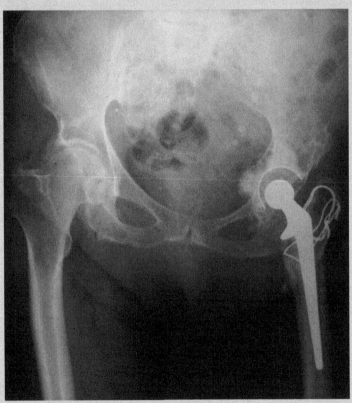

Fig. 9.12 Patient, 23 years after LFA, remains free of symptoms with activities suitable to her age. Left leg was lengthened 5 cm and leg-length discrepancy improved from 7 cm preoperatively to 2 cm postoperatively

Case 5

A 56-year-old patient with bilateral high dislocation. At the age of 23, in 1958, she had elsewhere intertrochanteric osteotomies on both hips (Figs. 9.13, 9.14, 9.15, 9.16, 9.17, 9.18, 9.19 and 9.20).

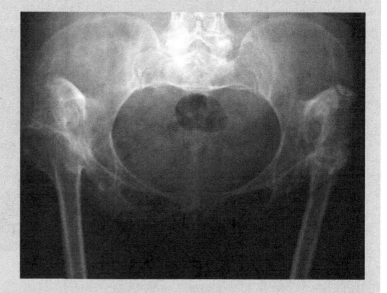

Fig. 9.13 Preoperative radiograph. The height of the dislocation was 7 cm on the left hip and 6 cm on the right

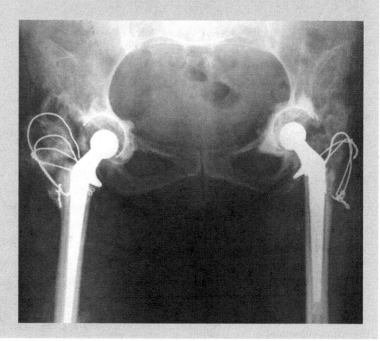

Fig. 9.14 LFAs were performed in 1991 with cotyloplasty technique, offset-bore cups and Harris CDH stems. Two years postoperatively, early loosening of the left stem, followed by isolated revision of the stem

Fig. 9.15 Radiograph
13 years after primary
replacement and 11 years
after revision of the left stem.
Note loosening of the right
cup and the left revised stem

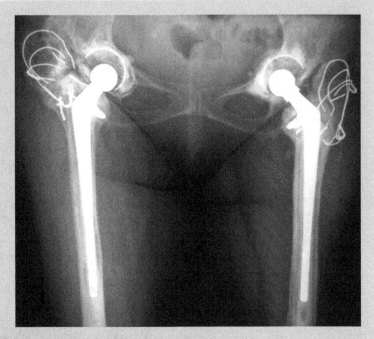

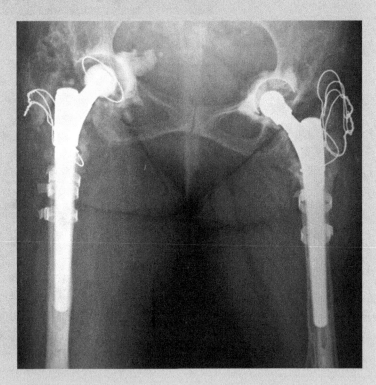

Fig. 9.16 Revision of both
components in the right hip
and rerevision of the stem in
the left was performed

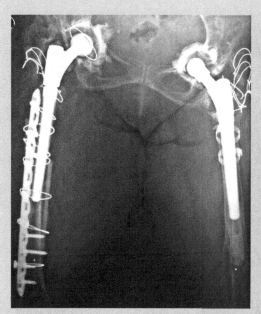

Fig. 9.17 Three years after revision, a periprosthetic fracture occurred on the right femur, fixed with plate and screws and strut allograft

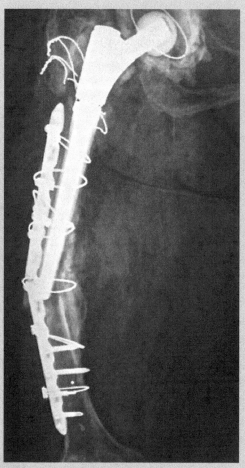

Fig. 9.18 The osteosynthesis failed (plate broke) 1 year after fixation, followed by a new revision of both components. Megaprosthesis (Stanmore, UK) and cortical strut allografts were used as a salvage procedure

Fig. 9.19 On the left hip, the cup was loose 2 years later and one more revision was performed, leading to peroneal nerve palsy

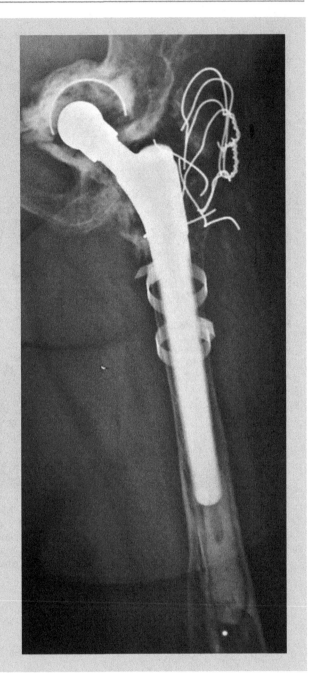

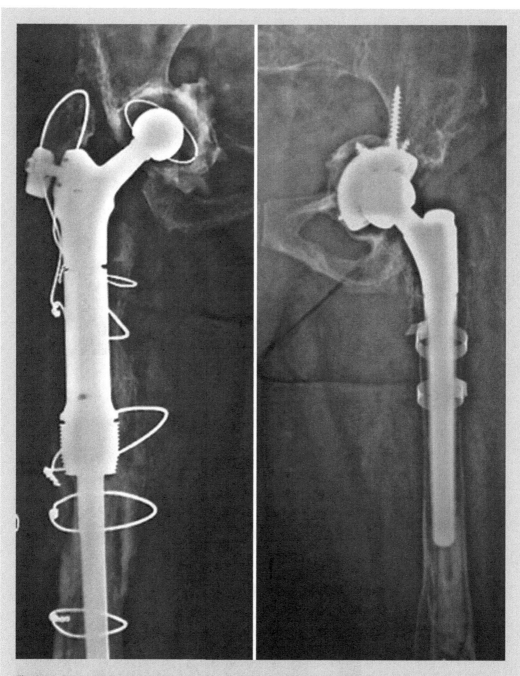

Fig. 9.20 Radiograph at the latest patient's follow-up examination 4 years after the last revision on right hip and 2 years on the left. In total, this patient had four operations on the right and four on the left hip. She is 77 years old and walks with difficulty using two crunches and has limited activity

Case 6

A 45-year-old patient with high dislocation on the left hip and idiopathic OA on the right. At the age of 17 (1962), she had Schanz osteotomy (Figs. 9.21, 9.22, 9.23 and 9.24).

Fig. 9.21 Radiograph taken when the patient was referred to us

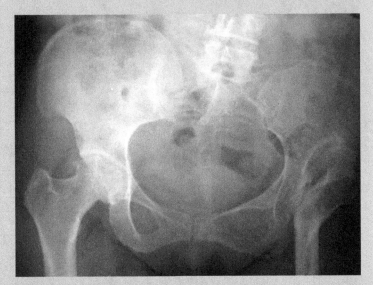

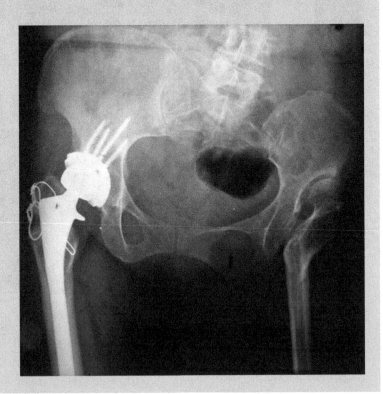

Fig. 9.22 She was first operated on the most painful right hip

Fig. 9.23 Radiograph
7 years after cementless THR
on the right hip and 5 years
after hybrid replacement on
the left

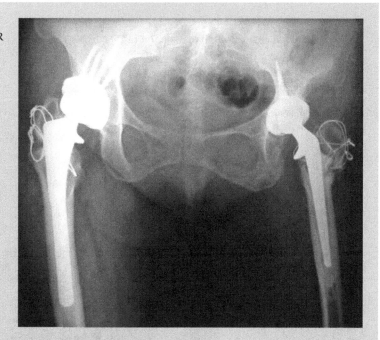

Fig 9.24 Left hip was
revised 10 years after primary
operation, and right after
16 years. This radiograph
was taken 16 years after the
first replacement of the right
hip. Patient walks with a
crutch on the left and has
limited level of activity

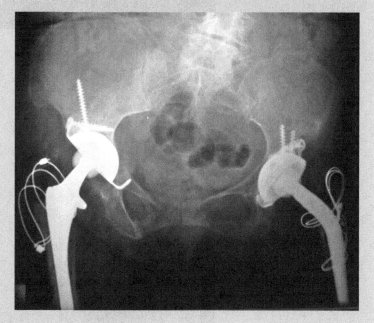

Case 7

A 71-year-old patient with high dislocation of the left hip. At the age of 40, in 1961, she had an intertrochanteric osteotomy (Figs. 9.25, 9.26, 9.27 and 9.28).

Fig. 9.25 Radiograph taken when the patient was referred to us. The height of the dislocation was 5 cm

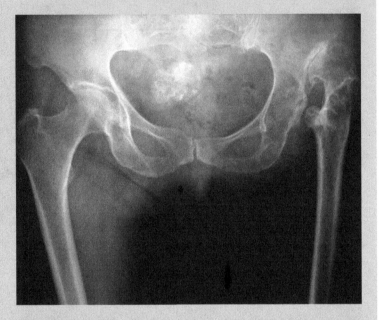

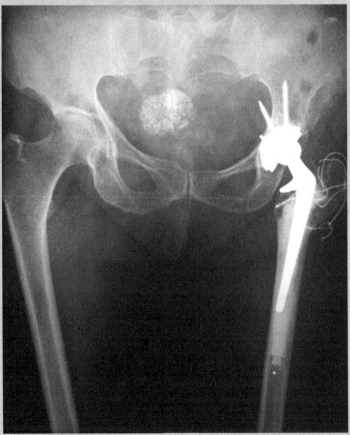

Fig. 9.26 Eight years after hybrid type of hip replacement with Harris-Galante cup and CDH cemented Harris stem

Fig. 9.27 Thirteen years postoperatively, wear of the polyethylene was noted

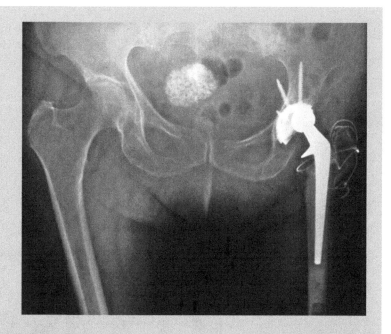

Fig. 9.28 The polyethylene was not available by the company and we were forced to use an alternative reconstruction method: we used cement to fix a new polyethylene in the original cup

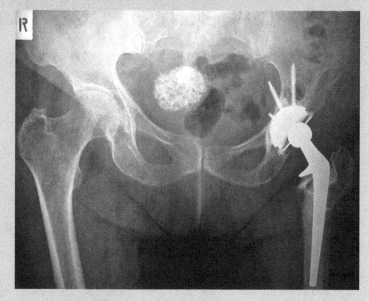

Case 8

Patient 54-year-old with bilateral low dis-location. At the age of 30, in 1969, she had a McMurray osteotomy on the right hip (Figs. 9.29, 9.30, 9.31 and 9.32).

Fig. 9.29 Preoperative radiograph

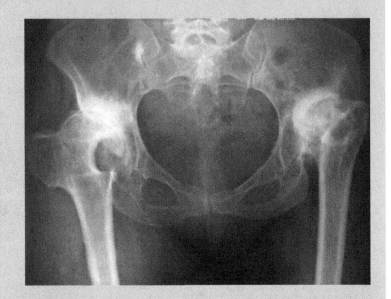

Fig. 9.30 Radiograph, 1 year after LFA on the right hip and hybrid-type arthroplasty on the left performed within 2 months. On the right hip, cotyloplasty was used. Note that intraoperatively the cup was medialised beyond the ilioischial line

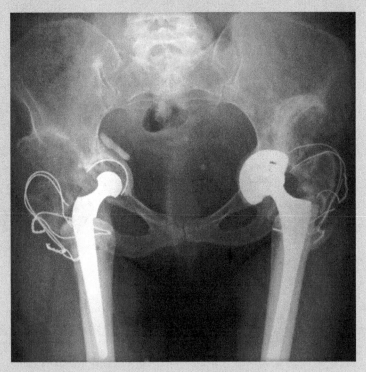

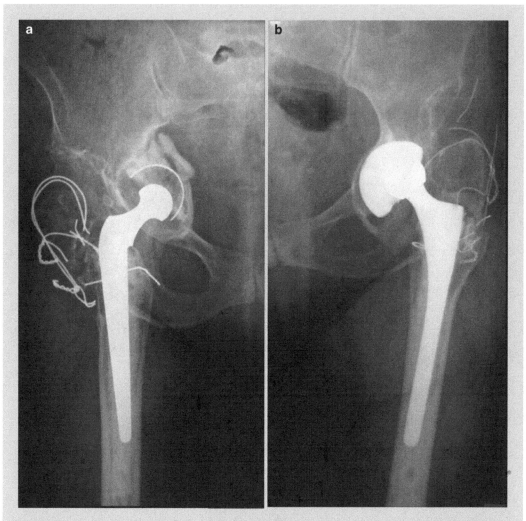

Fig. 9.31 Both hips required revision (**a**) 13 years the right hip and (**b**) 12 years the left after primary surgery

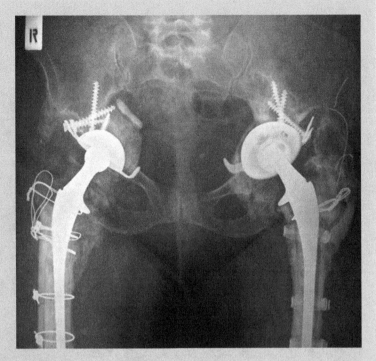

Fig. 9.32 Radiograph, 3 and 2 years after revision on the left and the right hip, respectively. The patient died from heart disease, at the age of 70, 16 years after the primary replacement

Case 9

Patient at the age of 61 with high dislocation on the left hip and low dislocation on the right.

In 1959, at the age of 27, she had elsewhere an intertrochanteric varus osteotomy on the right hip (Figs. 9.33, 9.34, 9.35 and 9.36).

Fig. 9.33 Preoperative radiograph. The height of the dislocation in the left hip was 10 cm (see also Fig. 6.6)

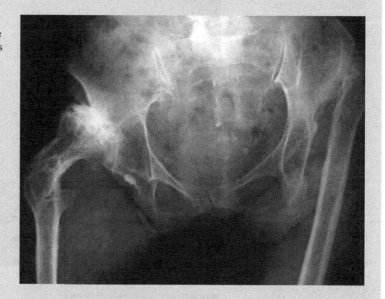

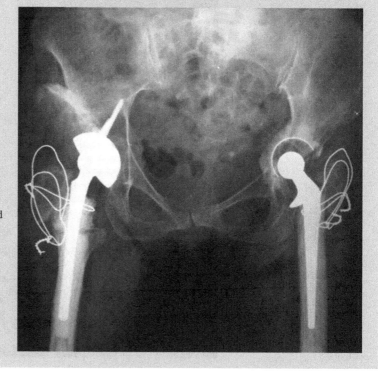

Fig. 9.34 She had bilateral THR within 1 month. On the right hip a hybrid-type arthroplasty was introduced (cementless Opti-Fix cup and a fixed with cement Opti-Fix stem No 0). The left hip was reconstructed with cotyloplasty, offset-bore cup and a cemented Harris CDH stem. Left leg was lengthened 5 cm, and leg-length discrepancy improved from 7 cm preoperatively to 2 cm after surgery

Fig. 9.35 Twelve years after primary replacement, left cup and both components on the right hip required revision because of loosening

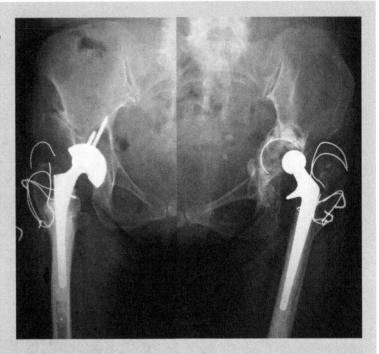

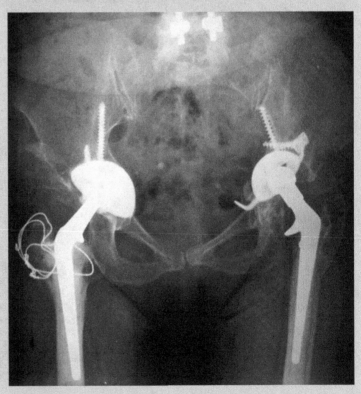

Fig. 9.36 Radiograph, 6 years after revision of the left hip and 5 after revision of the right. Patient at the age of 79 walks with two crutches and has limited activities

Case 10

Patient, age 60, with high dislocation of the right hip and idiopathic OA of the left. She had fusion of the right hip in another institution at the age of 14 (Figs. 9.37 and 9.38).

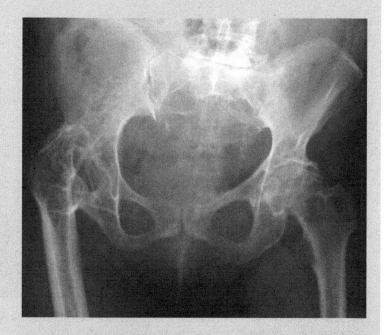

Fig. 9.37 Preoperative radiograph. Note that the right hip was fused with the extraarticular method of Brittain (see also Fig. 6.8)

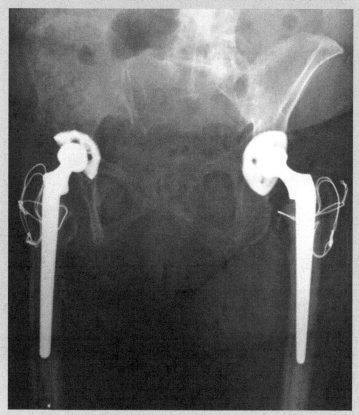

Fig. 9.38 THR was performed in both sides. The previous fusion of right hip made the reconstruction extremely difficult. Radiograph 14 years after THRs. Note the extreme vertical placement of the left cup in the attempt to achieve better bony coverage

Case 11
A 65-year-old patient with bilateral low dislocation had intertrochanteric osteotomy on the left hip at the age of 33 (1964) and on the right hip at the age of 44 (1975) (Figs. 9.39, 9.40 and 9.41).

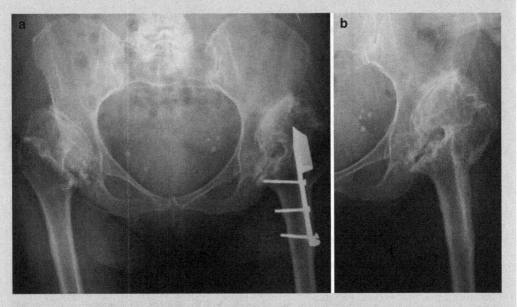

Fig. 9.39 (**a**) Note the great displacement of the femur on the left hip in the radiograph taken when the patient was referred to us. (**b**) Removal of the plate was performed before THR

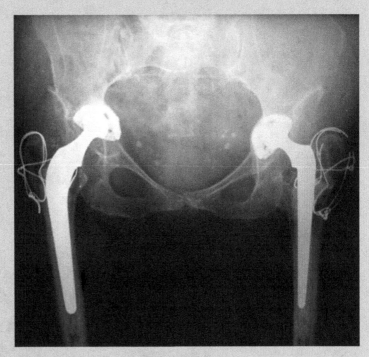

Fig. 9.40 Eight years after hybrid replacement of both hips. One year later exchange of the left liner was needed and after one more year revision of both components on the right hip

Fig. 9.41 Eleven years after primary replacement of both hips

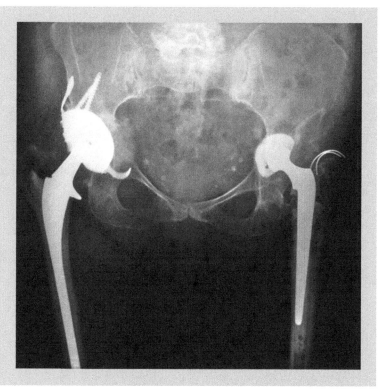

Timing for Revision

An artificial joint, especially in young patients with congenital hip disease (CHD), has the likelihood of revision after certain years of function. This may delay, even for 30 or more years, but sometimes will occur as patient remains active.

For that reason, the follow-up of patients with total hip replacement (THR) for a lifetime and revision at the appropriate time is of fundamental importance (Fig. 10.1). The decision for the time of revision belongs to the surgeon, in contrast to the decision for the primary replacement which is taken in consultation with the patient.

Revision of THR, previously performed for CHD, has a wide spectrum of difficulty. It can be from a rather simple isolated polyethylene insert exchange to the need for megaprosthesis.

If the patient has a proper follow-up and a severe wear of the usually small diameter polyethylene is detected early, an isolated exchange with concomitant femoral head exchange may suffice, provided that both components are stable and the polyethylene locking mechanism is intact (Figs. 11.27, 11.28, 11.29, 11.30 and 11.31). We have found, however, that companies do not always keep spare inserts for this exchange, thus the surgeon is forced to do a larger operation with consequences to the already defective bone stock and the economy.

Timely revision, before extensive bone destruction, may give to the patient several more years of a good quality's life (Figs. 10.2 and 10.3).

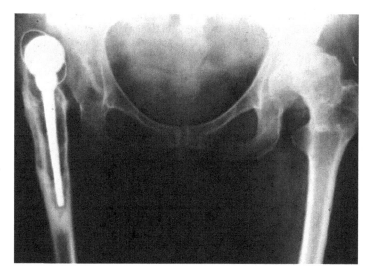

Fig. 10.1 This patient visited her surgeon 10 years after primary THR. The result is obvious: complete deboning of the acetabular component and gross loosening of the femoral stem with severe osteolysis in all zones. This catastrophic result could be avoided if the patient had a constant follow-up examination

G. Hartofilakidis et al., *Congenital Hip Disease in Adults*,
DOI 10.1007/978-88-470-5492-9_10, © Springer-Verlag Italia 2014

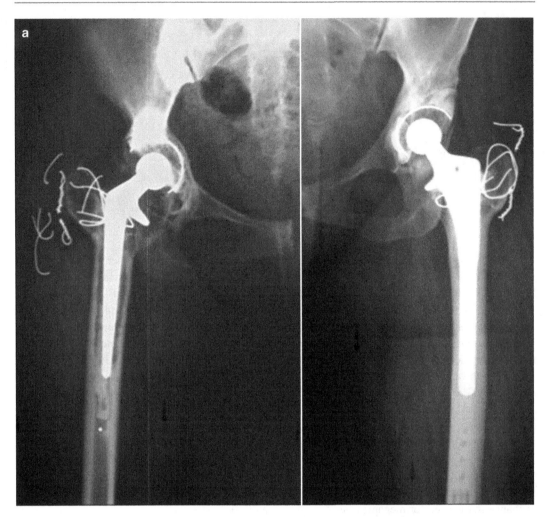

Fig. 10.2 Radiographs of a patient who had THR for high dislocation on the right hip and low dislocation on the left at the age of 25 years. (**a**) Fifteen years after surgery the left cup and both components on the right hip were loose and revised within 10 months. (**b**) Radiograph 9 years after revision. A Hilock (Symbios) cup was used for the revision of the left acetabulum. In the right side, an extended trochanteric osteotomy was necessary. For the revision of the acetabular component, a tantalum cup with XLPE (Zimmer) was used. For the femoral component a cemented revision-type stem (Elite Plus by DePuy) was utilised because the canal was too narrow for a cementless revision stem

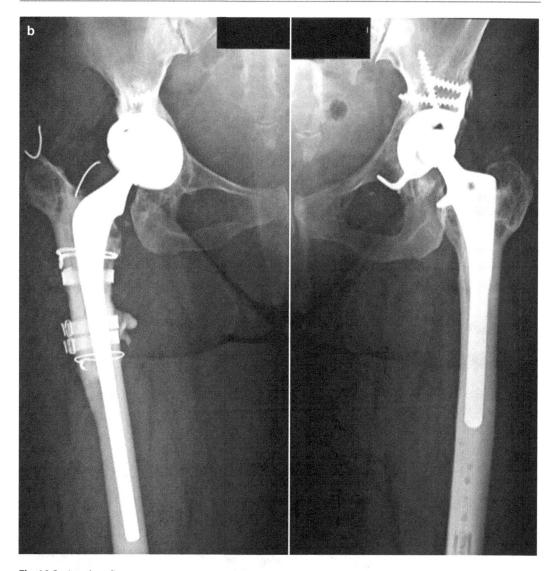

Fig. 10.2 (continued)

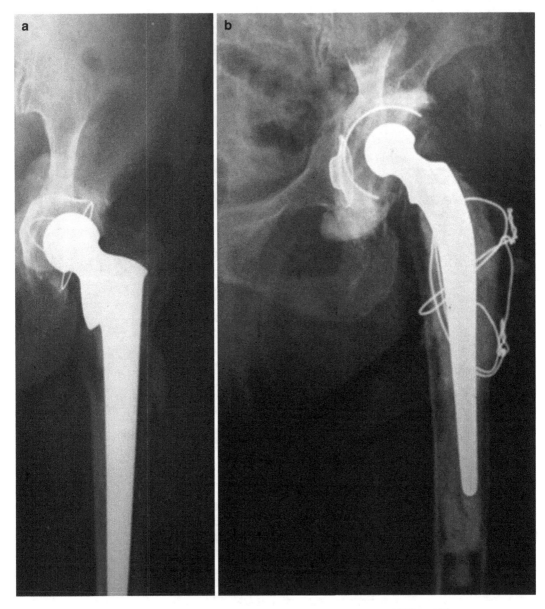

Fig. 10.3 This female patient had, at the age of 60, in another institution, a cemented THR. (**a**) Two years postoperatively both components were loose without extensive osteolysis. (**b**) Radiograph 24 years after revision with LFA

Cemented and cementless devices, used in the primary THR, have different failure mechanisms. Loosening remains the major problem of the cemented all-polyethylene acetabular components (Fig. 10.4). Radiographically the acetabular component is considered to be definitely loose when there is migration of >2 mm in the vertical or horizontal direction. In the presence of a circumferential radiolucent line, up to 2 mm, without migration or a change of the position, the component is considered as probably loose [1]. A probably loose cemented acetabular component does not need an argent revision. It can be survived for many more years (Fig. 10.5). Also, wear of the polyethylene of a cemented component, without progressive osteolysis, does not need forthwith revision. It can last for years without osteolysis and loosening (Fig. 10.6). On the other hand, cementless acetabular components present other potential causes of failure, mainly the possibility of early wear of the liner that has been documented in earlier designs (Fig. 10.7). We should be aware that the processes of wear and osteolysis are initially symptomless.

Modular metal-backed cementless prosthesis allows the liner to be exchanged, while leaving the stable metal shell in place. As it has been already said, the availability in the market of spare parts is a moral and legal obligation of the orthopaedic industry, which unfortunately is not always respected. This compels the surgeon to pursue other more complicated solutions which may be against the patient's health and public economics. Metal shell needs revision if more than 50 % of the shell surface is in contact with an area of osteolysis [2].

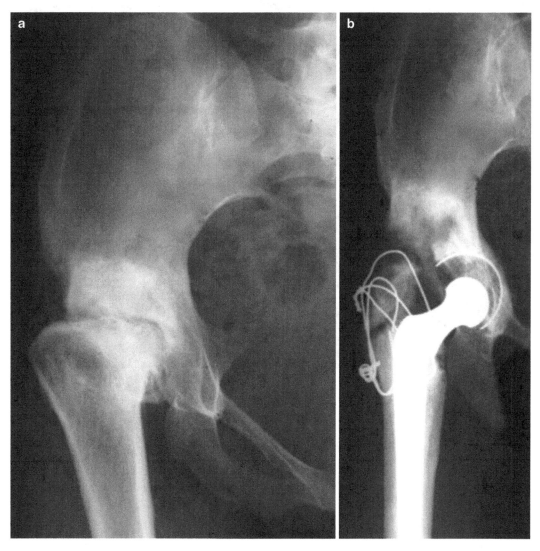

Fig. 10.4 Radiographs of a patient 26 years old with low dislocation of the right hip. (**a**, **b**) Pre- and postoperative radiographs after a Charnley LFA. (**c**, **d**) Radiographs 3 and 12 years after primary THR. Note the early loosening of the acetabular component indicating the need of revision (see also Fig. 11.11, 11.12, 11.13, 11.14 and 11.15)

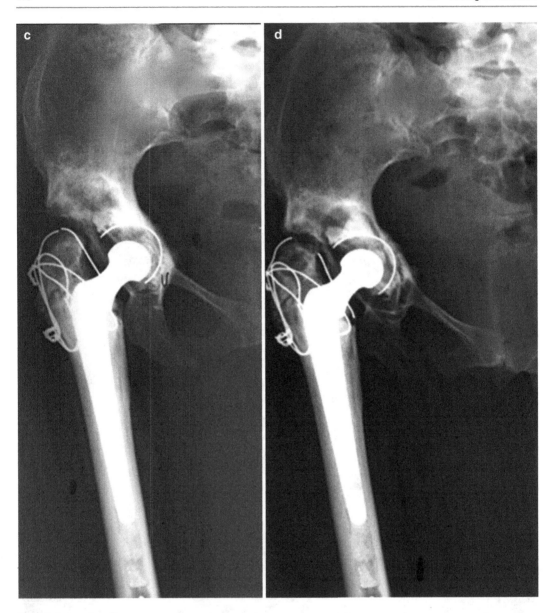

Fig. 10.4 (continued)

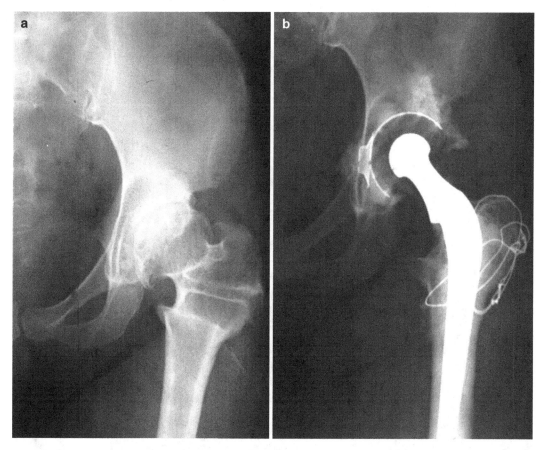

Fig. 10.5 Radiographs of a patient with dysplastic hip who had previously an intertrochanteric osteotomy. (**a**) Preoperative radiograph of the patient at the age of 37. (**b**) Two years after a LFA. (**c**) Twenty years after surgery. The acetabular component was characterised as probably loose. (**d**) Six years later the acetabular component remains probably loose without further deterioration

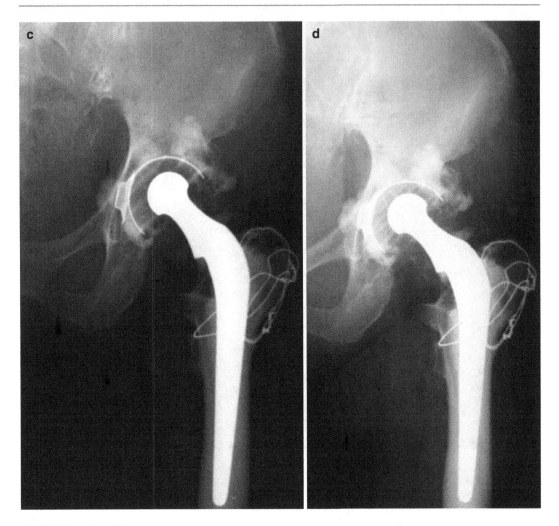

Fig. 10.5 (continued)

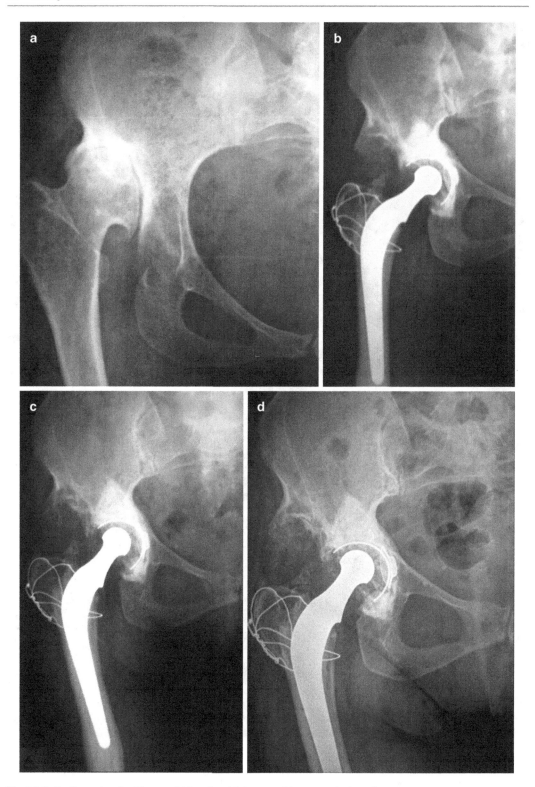

Fig. 10.6 Radiographs of a 30-year-old female with low dislocation in the right hip. (**a**) Preoperative radiograph. (**b**) Ten years after surgery. (**c**) Twenty-five years after surgery, there is significant wear of the polyethylene, without osteolysis or loosening. Further observation and no revision were decided. (**d**) For the next 8 years slight increase of wear permits further postponement of the revision

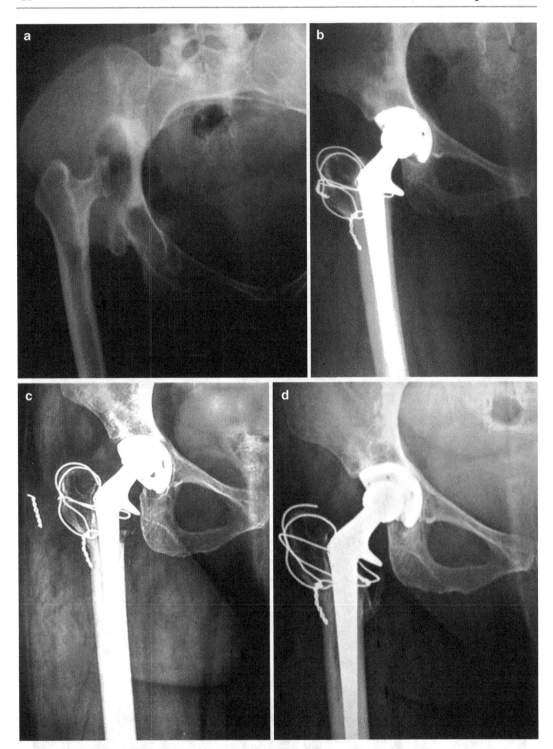

Fig. 10.7 A 38-year-old female with high dislocation of the right hip. (**a**) Preoperative radiograph. (**b**) Two years after hybrid THR. (**c**) Fourteen years postoperatively, the liner presented asymptomatic wear and was exchanged. (**d**) Radiograph 5 years after liner exchange and 19 years after primary replacement (see also Figs. 11.38, 11.39, 11.40, 11.41, 11.42, 11.43 and 11.44)

The decision to revise the femoral component, cemented or cementless, depends on the rate of progressive bone loss and loosening. The femoral component is classified as definitely loose when there is migration, change of position or subsidence of >2 mm. When there is only a continuous radiolucent line around the cement-bone or implant-bone interface, the component is classified as probably loose [3, 4]. A probably loose femoral component, without progressive osteolysis, may survive for years before revision is needed (Fig. 10.8).

Although revision operation is undesirable for the patients and has a significant financial burden, it can be successful if it is performed on time.

The senior author of this book (GH) has utilised the Charnley low-friction arthroplasty (LFA) techniques and implants, with good long-term results for failed hip replacements in patients with CHD without extensive bone loss (Fig. 10.9). Recent years, acetabular revision follows more current methods of reconstruction with porous or ultra-porous hemispherical cups.

Revision after failed primary THR in patients with CHD has additional technical difficulties, due to the already compromised anatomy and bone stock [5–8]. The acetabular

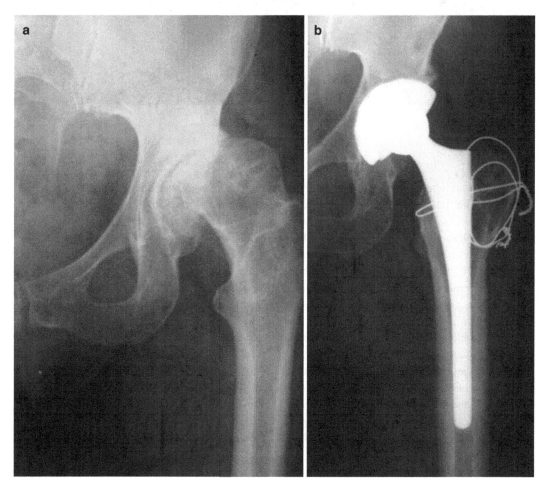

Fig. 10.8 Secondary osteoarthritis in a 53-year-old patient with dysplastic hip. (**a**) Preoperative radiograph. (**b**) Postoperative radiograph after a cementless THR. (**c**, **d**) Radiographs 7 and 12 years postoperatively, linear osteolysis around the femoral stem remains the same

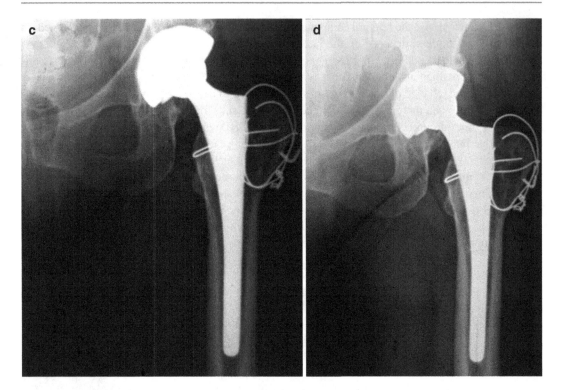

Fig. 10.8 (continued)

bone stock can be extremely deficient and the cortex of the femur thin. The presence of cement from the previous operation creates more difficulties. If there are areas at the femoral canal with well-fixed cement, it can be left in place using the technique so-called cement-in-cement, in order to avoid complications such as femoral fracture or cortex penetration [9].

In cases with no roof and/or walls to support the cup, we utilise porous metal augments, Busch-Schneider cages or cup-cage constructs depending on the extent of bone loss. Grit-blasted oblong cups with a hook and a side plate for additional screws have shown early loosening and are less popular today [10]. Intrapelvic protrusion of the acetabular

component is a severe complication mostly seen in cases with improper follow-up (Fig. 10.10).

Previous non-union of the greater trochanter predisposes for non-union after revision irrespectively of the method used to attach the trochanter to the host bone. In cases with narrow femoral medullary canal and absence of the metaphysis, we have encountered many difficulties to fit a cementless stem with the appropriate small diameter, and therefore a long cemented stem is used even in young patients (Fig. 10.11). When transfemoral and extended trochanteric osteotomies are utilised, the canal is straightened and "relaxed" allowing for the use of a cementless femoral component (Fig. 10.12). In severe unconstructible proximal femoral bone loss, proximal allograft

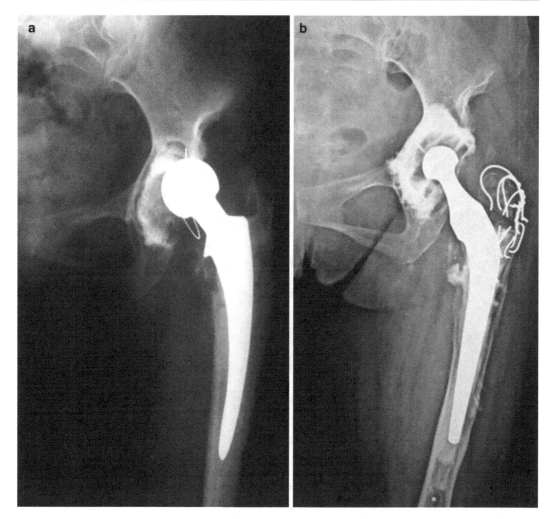

Fig. 10.9 Female patient who had elsewhere a Muller-type cemented THR for low dislocation at the age of 20. (**a**) Radiograph, 8 years postoperatively, depicts loosening of both components with moderate bone loss. (**b**) Twenty-five years after revision with LFA. Patient remains asymptomatic with full activity

prosthetic composites or tumour megaprostheses are the final solutions (Figs. 9.13, 9.14, 9.15, 9.16, 9.17, 9.18, 9.19 and 9.20) [11, 12].

The extent and type of pre-revision bone stock defects is believed to be the major determining factors of success in a revision of both the acetabular and femoral components. For the defects of the acetabulum, a simple and easy to remember classification system, is this of D'Antonio et al. [13] (Table 10.1). Similarly, for the defects of the femur, is the classification of Estok and Harris [14] (Table 10.2). Today, the most widely used classification system, for the assessment of defects of both acetabulum and femur, is that proposed by Paproski et al. [15, 16].

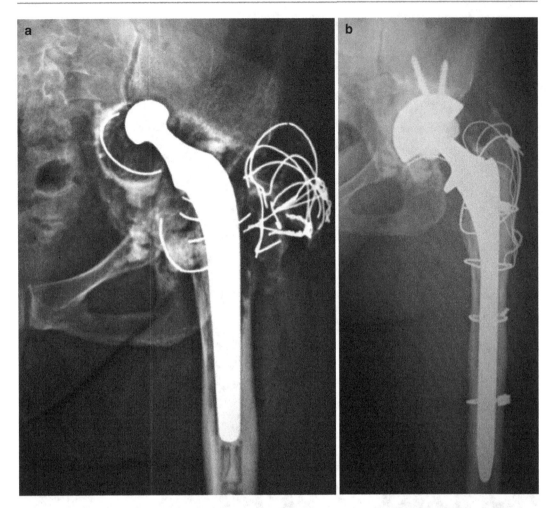

Fig. 10.10 (a) Severe intrapelvic protrusion without pelvic discontinuity 21 years after THR with cotyloplasty for low dislocation. Patient was not complied to follow-up examinations. (**b**) Six years after revision. Particulate bone grafting of the acetabular floor and a large hemispherical cup (ultra-porous tantalum) were utilised. At the femoral side a fully porous-coated stem was inserted after extended greater trochanter osteotomy

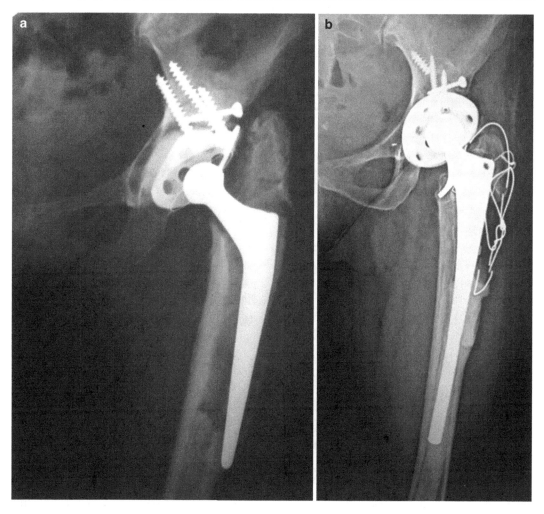

Fig. 10.11 (**a**) The lateral cortex of the proximal femur is missing in this referred case of a 33-year-old patient who had her primary THR 4 years ago. Revision was per-formed using cemented long femoral stem with distal fixation. (**b**) Radiograph, 19 years after revision

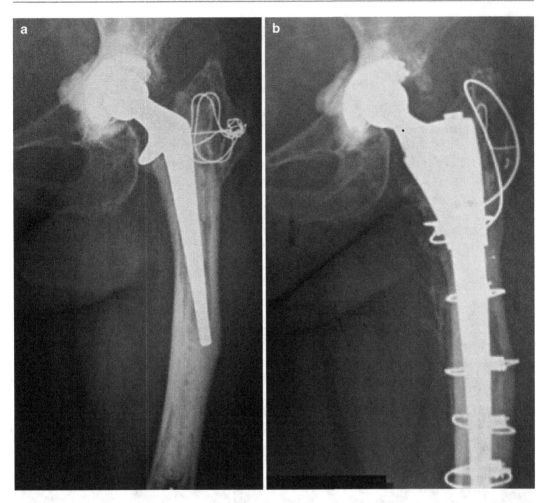

Fig. 10.12 (a) Extended trochanteric osteotomy in this particular case allowed for the use of a dual modular Wagner-type cementless stem (Profemur, Wright). (b) Follow-up radiograph at 6 years shows straightening of the femur along with femoral bone stock restoration. The figure-of-eight technique described by Ries was used to stabilise the greater trochanter

Table 10.1 The modified classification system of D'Antonio et al. for the pre-revision evaluation of acetabular bone defects

Types of acetabular bone defects	
A. Peripheral	1. Anterior wall
	2. Posterior wall
	3. Superior wall
B. Central (medial wall)	1. Attenuation (protrusion)
	2. Perforation
C. Combined	1. A3 + B1
	2. A3 + B2
	3. A1 + B2

Table 10.2 The classification system of Estok and Harris for the pre-revision evaluation of femoral bone defects

Types of femoral bone defects	
Grade I	Little or no cortical bone loss
Grade II	Moderate cortical bone loss
Grade III	Major bone loss

References

1. Hartofilakidis G, Karachalios T (2004) Total hip arthroplasty for congenital hip disease. J Bone Joint Surg Am 86-A(2):242–250

2. O'Brien JJ, Burnett RS, McCalden RW, MacDonald SJ, Bourne RB, Rorabeck CH (2004) Isolated liner exchange in revision total hip arthroplasty: clinical results using the direct lateral surgical approach. J Arthroplasty 19(4):414–423

3. Goetz DD, Smith EJ, Harris WH (1994) The prevalence of femoral osteolysis associated with components inserted with or without cement in total hip replacements. A retrospective matched-pair series. J Bone Joint Surg Am 76(8):1121–1129

4. Barrack RL, Mulroy RD Jr, Harris WH (1992) Improved cementing techniques and femoral component loosening in young patients with hip arthroplasty. A 12-year radiographic review. J Bone Joint Surg Br 74(3):385–389

5. Dearborn JT, Harris WH (2000) Acetabular revision after failed total hip arthroplasty in patients with congenital hip dislocation and dysplasia. Results after a mean of 8.6 years. J Bone Joint Surg Am 82-A(8):1146–1153

6. Hartofilakidis G, Stamos K, Karachalios T, Ioannidis TT, Zacharakis N (1996) Congenital hip disease in adults. Classification of acetabular deficiencies and operative treatment with acetabuloplasty combined with total hip arthroplasty. J Bone Joint Surg Am 78(5):683–692

7. Morag G, Zalzal P, Liberman B, Safir O, Flint M, Gross AE (2005) Outcome of revision hip arthroplasty in patients with a previous total hip replacement for developmental dysplasia of the hip. J Bone Joint Surg Br 87(8):1068–1072

8. Chougle A, Hemmady MV, Hodgkinson JP (2005) Severity of hip dysplasia and loosening of the socket in cemented total hip replacement. A long-term follow-up. J Bone Joint Surg Br 87(1):16–20

9. Duncan WW, Hubble MJ, Howell JR, Whitehouse SL, Timperley AJ, Gie GA (2009) Revision of the cemented femoral stem using a cement-in-cement technique: a five- to 15-year review. J Bone Joint Surg Br 91(5):577–582

10. Babis GC, Sakellariou VI, Chatziantoniou AN, Soucacos PN, Megas P (2011) High complication rate in reconstruction of Paprosky type IIIa acetabular defects using an oblong implant with modular side plates and a hook. J Bone Joint Surg Br 93(12):1592–1596

11. Sternheim A, Rogers BA, Kuzyk PR, Safir OA, Backstein D, Gross AE (2012) Segmental proximal femoral bone loss and revision total hip replacement in patients with developmental dysplasia of the hip: the role of allograft prosthesis composite. J Bone Joint Surg Br 94(6):762–767

12. Babis GC, Sakellariou VI, O'Connor MI, Hanssen AD, Sim FH (2010) Proximal femoral allograft-prosthesis composites in revision hip replacement: a 12-year follow-up study. J Bone Joint Surg Br 92(3):349–355

13. D'Antonio JA, Capello WN, Borden LS, Bargar WL, Bierbaum BF, Boettcher WG, Steinberg ME, Stulberg SD, Wedge JH (1989) Classification and management of acetabular abnormalities in total hip arthroplasty. Clin Orthop Relat Res 243:126–137

14. Estok DM, Harris WH (1994) Long-term results of cemented femoral revision surgery using second-generation techniques. An average 11.7-year follow-up evaluation. Clin Orthop Relat Res 299:190–202

15. Sporer SM, Paprosky WG (2003) Revision total hip arthroplasty: the limits of fully coated stems. Clin Orthop Relat Res 417:203–209

16. Paprosky WG, Perona PG, Lawrence JM (1994) Acetabular defect classification and surgical reconstruction in revision arthroplasty. A 6-year follow-up evaluation. J Arthroplasty 9(1):33–44

The long-term quality of life (QoL) of young female patients with congenital hip disease (CHD), especially those with low and high dislocation, radically improves after total hip replacement (THR) [1]. Before surgery these patients had severe limping, pain, body deformations in most of them and great leg-length discrepancy. They also had several psychological problems, such as anxiety and depression, even since their early childhood [2–8]. The severe disability had affected their lives in a fundamental way. Having usually experienced multiple and prolonged treatments since early childhood, they describe traumatic memories, especially those in the course of their development years.

The characteristic way these patients describe their mental and physical experiences is reflected in their letters included in our study on the QoL of patients of our registry [1]. This study was performed on 82 female patients, with low dislocation (67 hips) and high dislocation (48 hips), followed for a minimum of 12 years (12–37), and we concluded that THR radically improves QoL of these patients for a long period of time. Even patients who underwent several revisions had enjoyed pain relief and functional improvement for an appreciable period of time.

Representative cases are presented:

Case 1

A 37-year-old female with high dislocation of 7 cm on the left hip and low dislocation on the right (Fig. 11.1). She had no previ-

ous treatment. She was born in 1943. She was limping since infancy, but started to have pain in the right hip which had low dislocation, approximately at the age of 25. In 1981, at the age of 40, she had a Charnley low-friction arthroplasty (LFA), initially on the right hip (Fig. 11.2) and 5 months later on the left with cotyloplasty (Fig. 11.3). Preoperatively, right leg-length was 70 cm and the left 65 cm. Postoperatively, the leg-lengths were 72 cm right and 69 cm left. Eight years after surgery both components of the left hip were revised because of loosening (Fig. 11.4). Six years later, the left femur was fractured and the stem was rerevised (Fig. 11.5). The left cup was also rerevised because of wear, 22 years after revision (Fig. 11.6). Right hip was revised because of loosening, 18 years after primary replacement.

In total, this patient had three revisions on the left hip and one on the right (Fig. 11.7). At the latest follow-up examination, 32 years after primary surgery, the patient, at the age of 72, stated that she was partially satisfied from her hip problem. Letter sent:

I was born in a small Greek village during the 2nd World War. My parents, poor and illiterate, had to raise 4 daughters. My mother was treating me badly. She was referring to me as calling me a "crippled" and "half person". When others were listening, these words were hurting me more. I was ridiculed by the other children in school. When the teacher of gym wanted to put me out not to be tired I was crying.

Since I was 12 years old I started working as a housemaid in several houses. When I started feeling pain, at the age of 25, my life became unbearable. I had to work hard while in pain and great difficulties even getting around. I was 38 when I had my hips operated.

The result was outstanding. Pain was gone and stopped feeling useless. For the next 15 years, I was feeling very good, getting around as a normal person. I had no pain and I was barely limping. After that I had undergone three more operations on my left hip and one operation on my right hip.

I am now 72 years old and all I want is a life without pain. I have faith in God and in my surgeon and I believe that everything will go well.

Fig. 11.1 Preoperative radiograph

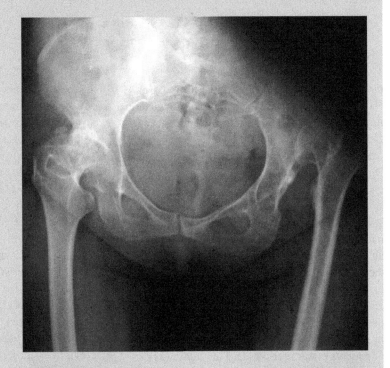

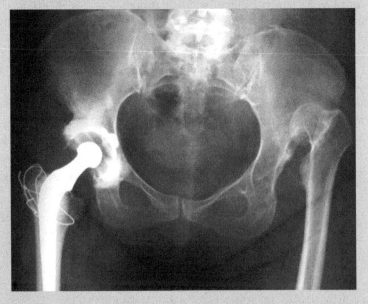

Fig. 11.2 Radiograph after LFA on the right hip

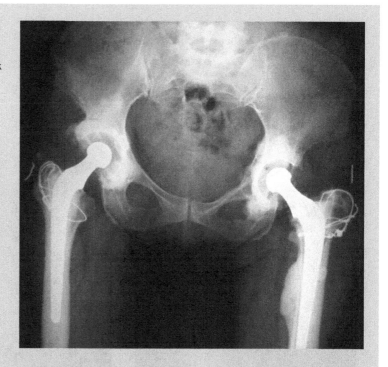

Fig. 11.3 Radiograph taken 5 years after LFA on both hips. Note the escape of cement from the inner cortex of the left femur due to penetration during surgery

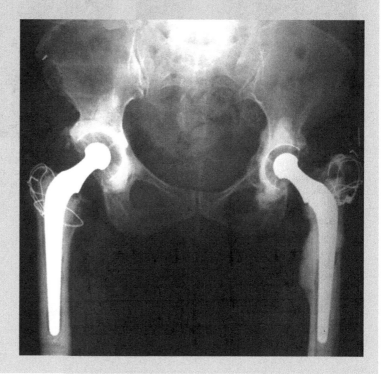

Fig. 11.4 Eight years after primary operations, the left hip needed revision because of loosening

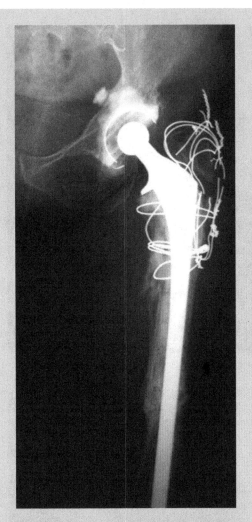

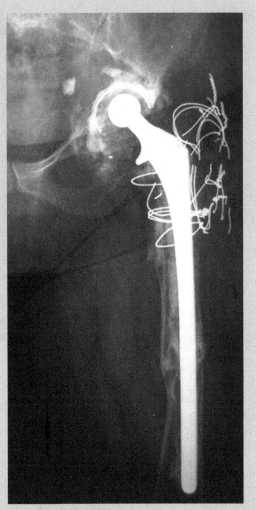

Fig. 11.5 Two years after revision of the left hip, performed because of a periprosthetic fracture of the femur. Abundant wires are due to the failure of removal of the wires used at the primary replacement. Note the union of the fracture at the middle of the femur

Fig. 11.6 Wear of the polyethylene, severe osteolysis and pelvic dissociation required a rerevision of acetabular component that was performed 22 years after previous revision

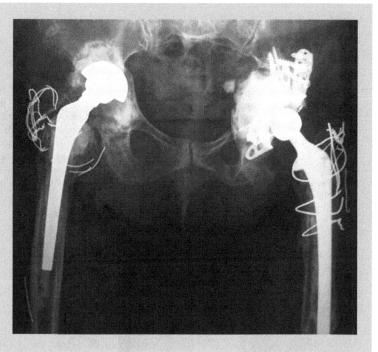

Fig. 11.7 Final radiograph, 32 years after primary THRs. The left hip has been revised three times and the right one

Case 2

This patient with low dislocation of the left hip had a THR at the age of 20, in another institution. Eight years later, revision was needed because of loosening of both components (Fig. 11.8). A LFA with cotyloplasty was used (Fig. 11.9). Since that time (25 years) this patient is symptomless with normal activity (Fig. 11.10). Letter sent:

> I was born in a village in Kalavryta. We were a big family (7 children). The parents were illiterate and poor. I was operated at the age of 4. I kept limping. My childhood was a life of torment. My mother was calling me names. She was calling me an invalid, a broken one, a limping creature. She was cursing me many times. She would tell me no man is going to love me. She and my older brother made me feel useless. I had arthroplasty at 20 and a second one at 28. My life changed. I don't feel useless anymore. My friends tell me that nothing shows when I walk. I met my husband and we were married in 1996. Now we have a 15 year old son and we are a happy family.

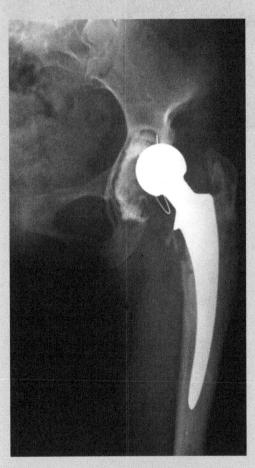

Fig. 11.8 Seven years after cemented, Muller-type THR. The need of revision is obvious

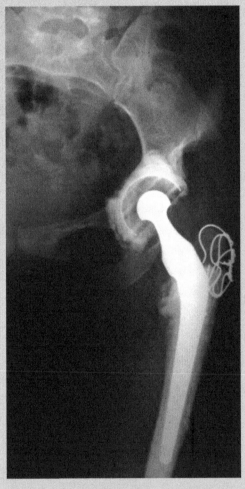

Fig. 11.9 One year after revision with LFA. Note the fibrous union of the trochanter

Fig. 11.10 Latest follow-up radiograph, 25 years after revision. Patient remains symptomless without limping

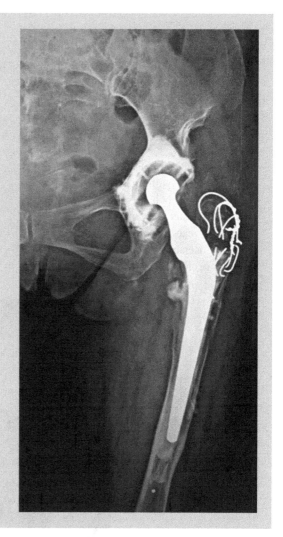

Case 3

This patient was born in 1961 with bilateral CHD. There is no information about the type of conservative treatment she had at the age of 2, followed by an operation on the right hip at the age of 3. She was first seen by us at the age of 26 with low dislocation on the right hip and dysplasia on the left (Fig. 11.11). She had severe pain and limping from the right hip. A Charnley LFA with cotyloplasty was performed on the right hip (Fig. 11.12) and 3 years later a varus osteotomy on the left (Fig. 11.13).

Eleven years after primary replacement, the right acetabular component was revised because of loosening (Fig. 11.14). A new

revision of acetabular component was needed after 13 years (Fig. 11.15). Femoral component remains stable for 25 years. Letter sent:

> I was born with a dislocation in my right hip. At the age of one and a half they put me in plaster for one year, and later I was operated. I kept limping. My childhood and teenage life were very difficult with many complexities and insecurities. I was feeling like a child of an inferior God. I took the decision to have an arthroplastic surgery at the age of 29. The result was very good. I developed faith for myself and I felt security. I was married and had a boy that became the joy and purpose of my life. Even though in 1994 it was necessary to be operated again, now I am fully active with a normal life. I am very pleased.

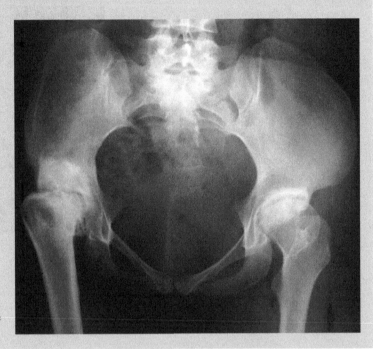

Fig. 11.11 Radiograph at the age of 26

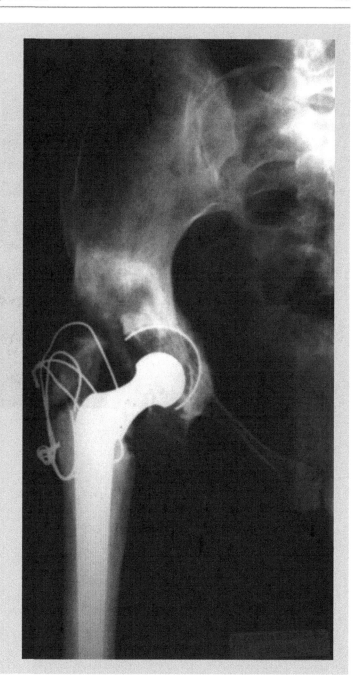

Fig. 11.12 Postoperative radiograph after LFA on the right hip. Fibrous union of the trochanter

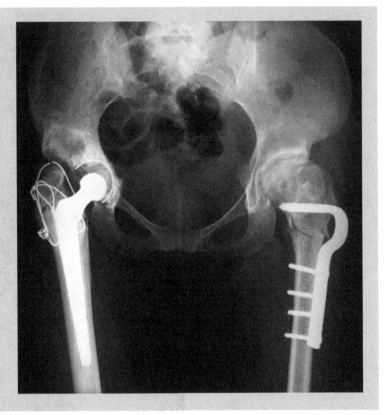

Fig. 11.13 Three years later a varus osteotomy was performed on the left hip

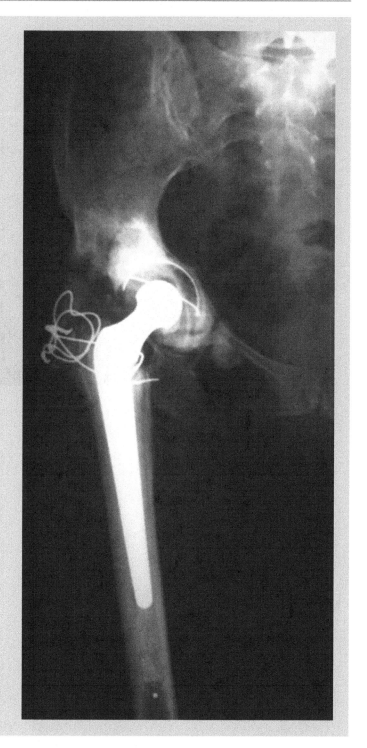

Fig. 11.14 Radiograph after revision of the right acetabular component, 11 years after primary replacement

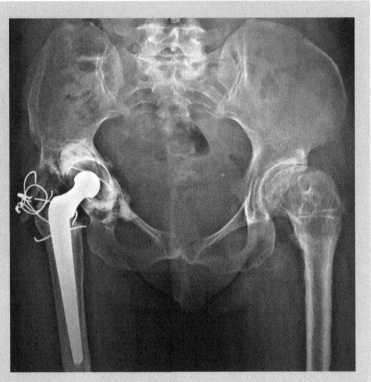

Fig. 11.15 Loosening of the revised acetabular component after 13 years from revision

Case 4

A 46-year-old female with bilateral high dislocation. She was born in 1942. The height of the dislocation was 8 cm in the right and 7 cm in the left hip (Fig. 11.16). She had no previous treatment. She started having pain at the age of 35. The preoperative leg-length was 71 cm right and 70 cm left and the postoperative 75 cm right and 75 cm left.

Cemented THRs with cotyloplasty technique were performed within 1 month (Fig. 11.17). Patient remained pain-free and without limping for the next 24 years (Fig. 11.18). Letter sent:

I was born in a small village of Macedonia. I had dislocation in both hips. My life was an Odyssey. In the school the children were making fun of me that I was so different because of the pelvic deformity and my movements was bothering me. I became melancholic and withdrawn. At the age of 9 I had two operations in my right hip and one in the left. I was still limping. Later I started having pains and my life became more difficult. I was avoiding relationships with the other sex for fear of rejection. When I had the arthroplasties in my hips I was at 47. My life changed. I did not have limping and pains. The shape of my body changed. I look at the mirror and I don't believe my eyes. People who knew me did not recognize me. Twenty-four years are gone since I was operated. I have a normal life with some anxiety for the future. My doctor puts me at ease saying that for whatever happens there is a solution.

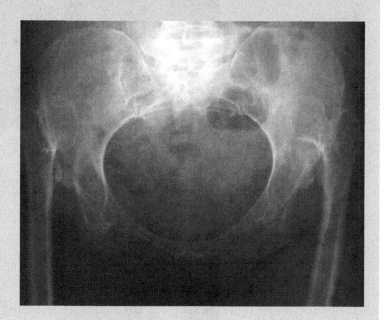

Fig. 11.16 Preoperative radiograph

Fig. 11.17 One year postoperatively

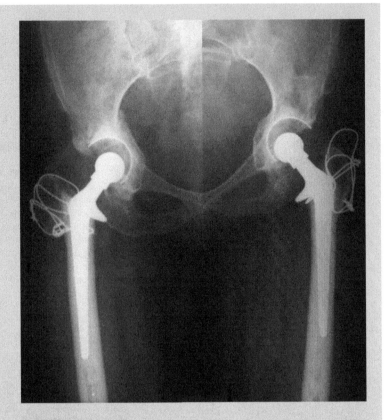

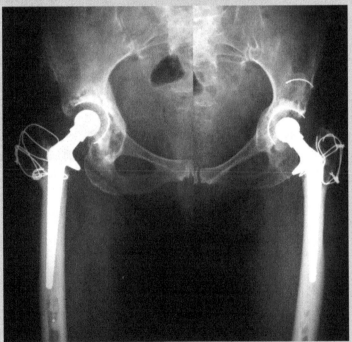

Fig. 11.18 Latest radiograph, 24 years after primary operations. Note the wear of the offset-bore acetabular components without significant osteolysis

Case 5

Patient with bilateral CHD. She was born in 1964. At the age of 2, she was treated conservatively (no more information about the type of treatment is available). She was first seen by us at the age of 25 (Fig. 11.19). She had high dislocation of 7 cm on the right hip and low dislocation on the left. Preoperatively, leg-length was 76 cm right and 82 cm left and postoperatively 80 and 82 cm, respectively. LFA was performed in both hips within 1 month. Cotyloplasty technique was used in the right hip (Fig. 11.20). Fifteen years later, the left acetabular component and after 1 year both components on the right hip were revised (Fig. 11.21). The patient had one more revision 5 years later of the right cup. Twenty-four years after primary hip replacements, the patient is asymptomatic and has normal activities (Fig. 11.22). Letter sent:

> I was born with dislocation in both hips. At age 2 half of my body was placed in plaster for about 6 months. I remember that I was crying and striking on the plaster as if wanted to break it. When I went to school I was getting upset when I heard different comments, like "Why they put this school girl in the parade" or "What a shame, such a beautiful girl moving like a boat". At the age of 25 (in 1989) I was operated because I had pain and was limping a lot. After the operation I felt that I was reborn. I was married, I had 2 daughters by Caesarian. For 15 years I was at my best. Later on it was necessary to be operated again twice in my right, and once in my left hip. Now I am very well. I am pleased and hopeful for the future.

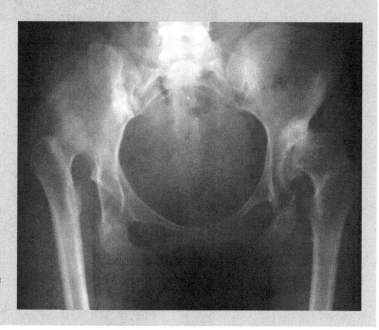

Fig. 11.19 Patient at the age of 25. Preoperative radiograph

Fig. 11.20 Radiograph
1 year postoperatively

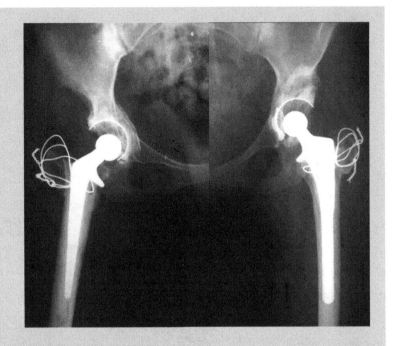

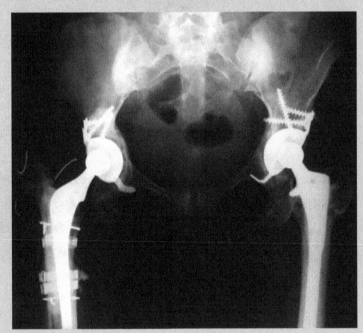

Fig. 11.21 Radiograph
17 years after primary hip
replacements. The cup on the
left hip was revised 2 years
previously. On the right hip
both components were revised
1 year previously

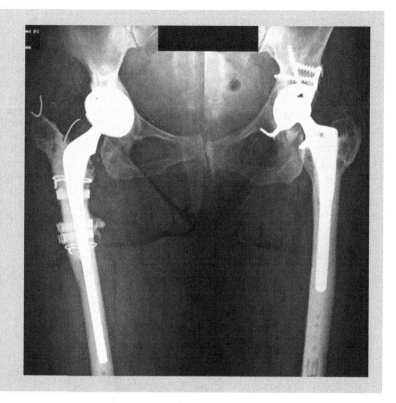

Fig. 11.22 Radiograph performed on the latest follow-up examination, 24 years after primary intervention (see also Fig. 10.2)

Case 6

This patient was born in 1949. She was 2 years old when she was treated conservatively for bilateral CHD. At the age of 19, radiograph showed low dislocation on the right hip and dysplasia on the left. Patient had mild limping from the right hip (Fig. 11.23). At the age of 40, she had severe pain and severe limping (Fig. 11.24). She had a LFA first on the right hip in combination with cotyloplasty and 20 days later on the left (Fig. 11.25). Twenty-four years after surgery, at the age of 64, the patient is asymptomatic and is fully active (Fig. 11.26). Letter sent:

I was born with dislocation in both hips. At the age of 2 I had some therapy with plaster. I remember that I was limping since I was a child and I started to have pains after the age of 20. When I was very young the other children were calling a "lame" that was hurting me and I was breaking out sobbing to my parents who were trying to comfort me. I was growing up agonizing, worrying with disappointments. I could not go places with buses or even a taxi. I delayed to be operated because I was afraid. In the end I decided when I was 40. Since then my life changed. Twenty-four years are gone. I am living normally, I am going places like the other people and I am happy.

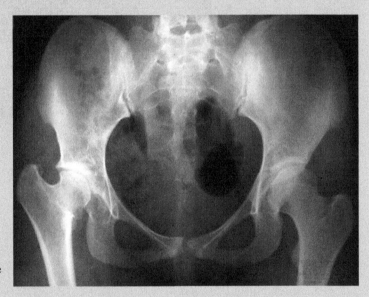

Fig. 11.23 Radiograph at the age of 19

Fig. 11.24 Preoperative radiograph when the patient was 40 years old

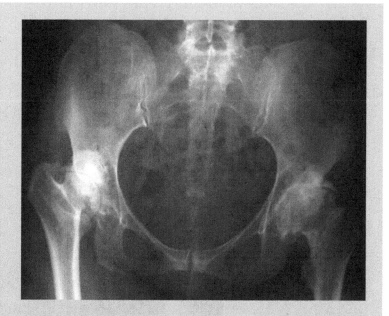

Fig. 11.25 Postoperative radiograph. For the reconstruction of the right hip, the cotyloplasty technique and the offset-bore acetabular component were used

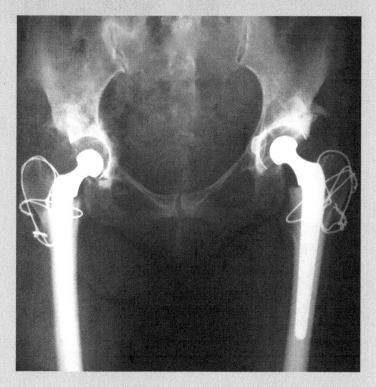

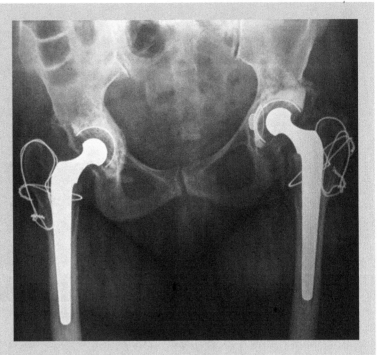

Fig. 11.26 Radiograph of the latest follow-up examination, 24 years after primary THRs

Case 7

A 31-year-old female born in 1959 with bilateral high dislocation. At the age of 2, she had an unsuccessful treatment. The height of the dislocation was 9 cm in both hips (Fig. 11.27). Preoperative leg-length was 71 cm in both sides and 74 cm postoperatively. Hybrid THR was performed on both hips within 18 days. Left hip was dislocated 20 days after surgery reduced under general anaesthesia (Fig. 11.28) and remained stable since that time (Fig. 11.29). Fourteen years after surgery liners of both hips were exchanged, at the same time because of progressive wear (Fig. 11.30).

At the latest follow-up examination, 23 years after primary replacements and 9 years after liner exchange, the patient remains without pain or limping living a normal life (Fig. 11.31). Letter sent:

> I was born in a small village near Amaliada. I had dislocation in both hips. My God, why? Since I was very young I was in adventures with different unsuccessful therapies. Fortunately, I had a great support from my parents. I was a single child. I was feeling being different, but I was trying not to stay away from social life. My psychological condition became worse after 30 when I started having pains. I was not late to decide for an operation. The change was enormous. My body became straight; it became 5 cm higher. Some people spoke of a miracle. I believe it. For any of those who have the same problem I have an advice: willingness and faith to improve their life, a right choice of a doctor, not only a competent scientist, but a human being too, and support from the family.

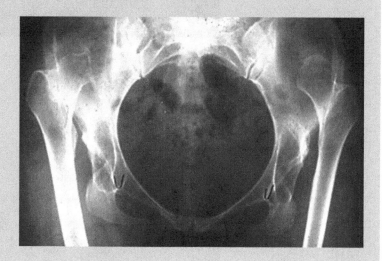

Fig. 11.27 Preoperative radiograph (see also Fig. 4.12)

Fig. 11.28 For the reconstruction the hybrid method was utilised. Dislocation of the left hip 20 days after surgery reduced under general anaesthesia

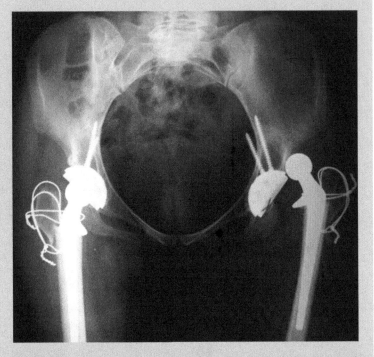

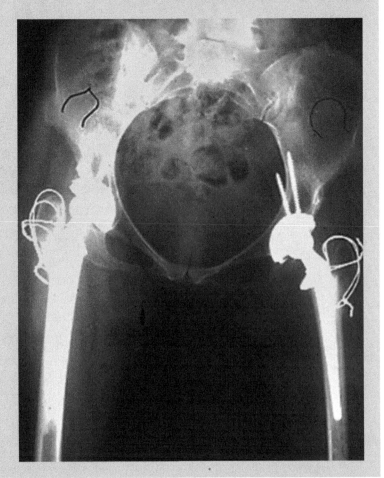

Fig. 11.29 One year postoperatively both hips remained stable

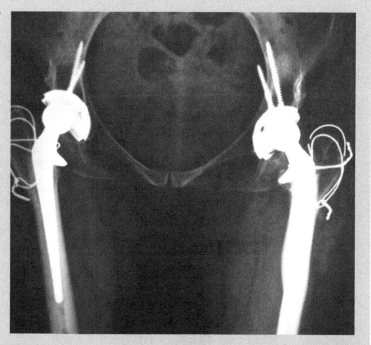

Fig. 11.30 Advanced wear of both polyethylene liners 14 years after surgery. Simultaneous bilateral liners' exchange was performed

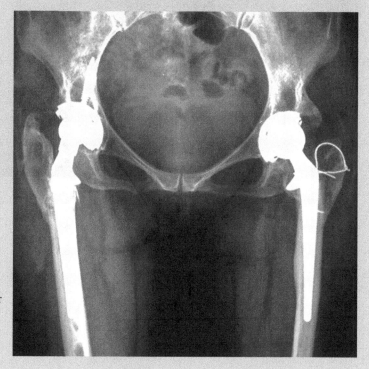

Fig. 11.31 Radiograph at the latest follow-up, 24 years after primary surgery. In the meantime exchange of both liners was performed due to wear

Case 8

A 42-year-old patient, born in 1951, with high dislocation of 4 cm in the right hip and low dislocation in the left (Fig. 11.32). She had no previous treatment. She was limping since infancy, but started to have pain in the left hip at the age of 35. Preoperative leg-length was 81 cm right and 82 cm left and postoperative 82 and 81 cm, respectively. Hybrid THR was performed in both hips within 1 month (Fig. 11.33). Twenty years after surgery, patient remains without pain having a mild limping only (Fig. 11.34). She has been fully active. Letter sent:

> I was born with dislocation in both hips, in a village in Evros. I began realizing it in my

childhood, at about 5 years old, when I was playing outside and I was getting easily tired. My parents were late to worry and visit different doctors in our nearby own. The doctors recommended operation, but my parents were afraid and were postponing. In the school I was participating in all activities, but I remember, with a great effort because I was getting easily tired. I was a good learner and a social individual. I had many female and male friends. In my teenage years I was, both, successful and unsuccessful as a woman. I worked as an administrative employee for 36 years and I had a happy family with 2 children and one most beautiful granddaughter. In the last 20 years when I had my hip operations my life has changed. Now I am a normal individual.

Fig. 11.32 Preoperative radiograph

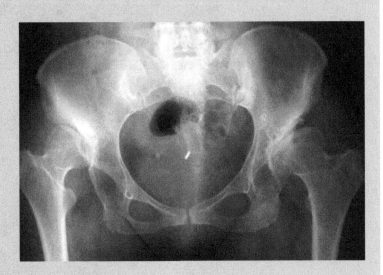

Fig. 11.33 The hybrid method was utilised. One year after surgery

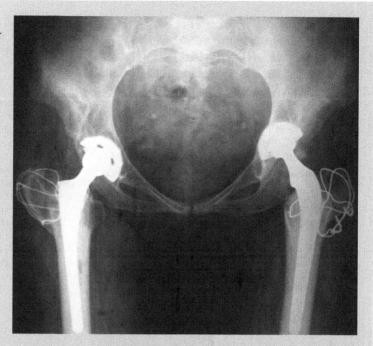

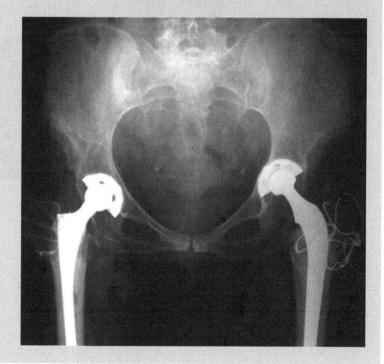

Fig. 11.34 Radiograph 20 years after THRs

Case 9

A 41-year-old patient born in 1952 with low dislocation in the left hip (Fig. 11.35). At the age of 8 years, she was operated in a children hospital. There is no information about the type of operation she had. She was limping since childhood and from the age of 25 she started having pain. Preoperative leg-length was 72 cm left and 74 cm right and postoperative 74 cm in both sides. She had a hybrid-type THR at the age of 41 (Fig. 11.36). She remains without pain and only mild limping 20 years after surgery (Fig. 11.37). Letter sent:

> I was born in Zakynthos. I had dislocation in the left hip. I was limping a lot and at the age of 9 they brought me to a hospital in Athens. I stayed alone for many months. My parents, poor country people, did not have to pay even for the fare to come and see me. I was feeling deserted. I suffered a lot. I had a large plaster up to the knee and a nail below the knee. After 6 months I was operated. When I came out of the plaster, plaster again from the waist down for another 6 months. When I came out of the plaster I had two small, atrophic feet and I learned from the beginning to walk like the babies. All these I remember after 50 years and I sob my heart out. Now 20 years are gone since I had the surgery. I have no pain and I walk almost without limping. I have a family with 2 children and I live a normal life. I always have the fear that I may have another surgery, but I am trying to put it out of my mind. I am so much close to my doctor that I would not have anyone else to take care of me.

Fig. 11.35 Preoperative radiograph

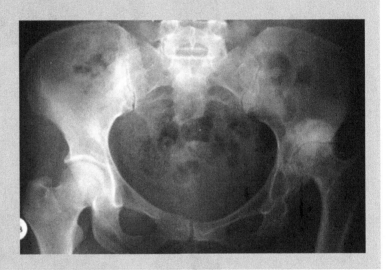

Fig. 11.36 One year after hybrid hip replacement

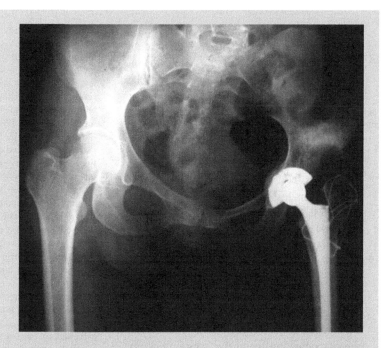

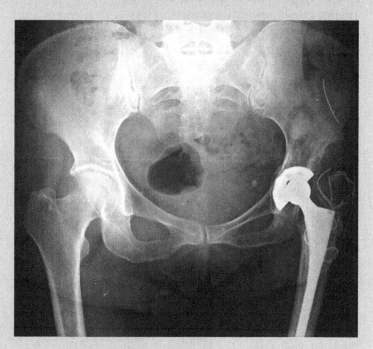

Fig. 11.37 The latest radiograph, 20 years postoperatively

Case 10

This patient born in 1951 with high dislocation of 7 cm on the right hip and low dislocation on the left. She had no treatment at infancy. She started having pain in the left hip at the age of 30 (Figs. 11.38 and 11.39). She was operated at the age of 43, first on the right hip and a month later on the left. Hybrid THR was used in both hips (Fig. 11.40). Preoperative leg-length was 66 cm right and 70 cm left and postoperatively 71 and 72 cm, respectively. Two years after surgery, left hip developed late infection (Fig. 11.41) which was treated by a specialised physician with antibiotics for 2 years. Nine years later, the stem on the left hip was broken (Fig. 11.42) and there followed by revision of both components. In the right hip PE was exchanged because of wear 13 years after primary replacement (Fig. 11.43). The patient remains symptom-free at the latest follow-up, 19 years after she was first operated (Fig. 11.44). Letter sent:

> I was born smiling from the first moment, without knowing that I have two hips with

dislocations and that they were to bring me many tears and pains. I remember my parents taking me to the doctors, examinations, X-Ray pictures, without a single good result. I was left to limp and with many psychological problems. In the school no child wanted to be with me in school events, gymnastics, marching by events etc. They were thinking of me as a second class child. It was very painful to me. I still remember and cry. Later I started travelling abroad for my problem of the hips without any good results. When I became 30 I started having pains and my life became more difficult. I could stand it, but every time it was worse. I came to the point to "crawl" and be unable to take care of myself. I had unbearable pains. In 1994 I was already 43 when I met my doctor. From the first moment he gave me hope, security and confidence. We did the arthroplasties and my life changed. I did not have pains anymore and I did not limp. I became a normal human like all the others. I was not afraid that my daughter could feel ashamed to have a lame mother. Ten years after the operation I had some problems because of complications that were taken care with success. Now I am well, I enjoy life and I thank God and my doctor for giving me the gift of the quality of life.

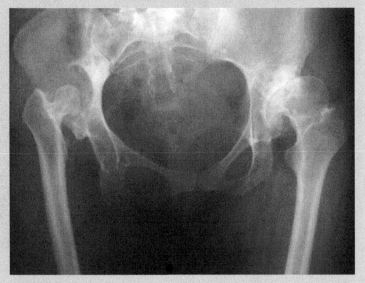

Fig. 11.38 Radiograph of the patient at the age of 34

Fig. 11.39 Radiograph when the patient was 43 years old. Note the absorption of the right femoral head

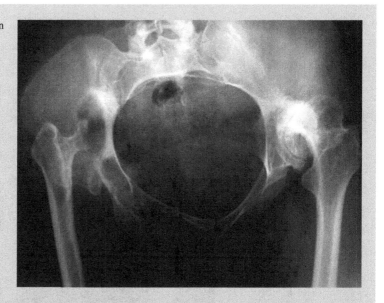

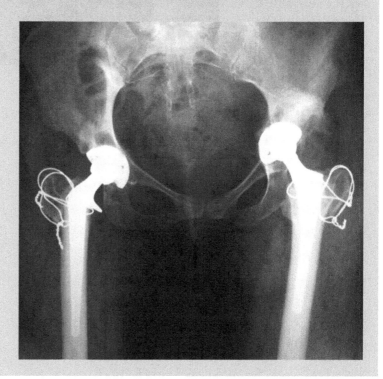

Fig. 11.40 The hybrid method was used bilaterally. Postoperative radiograph

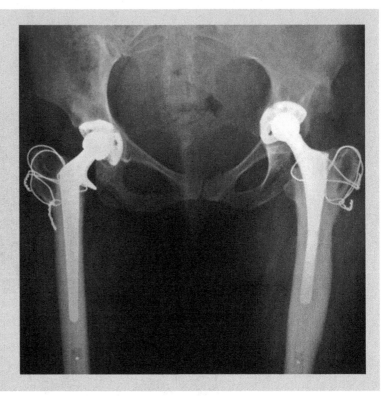

Fig. 11.41 Two years later postoperative infection was developed on the left hip treated with antibiotics

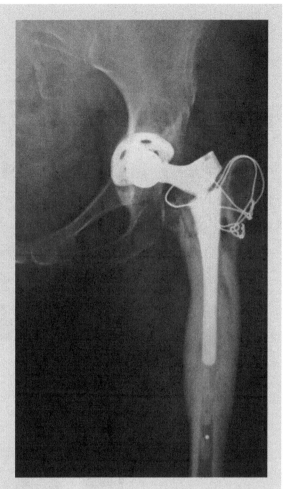

Fig. 11.42 Left stem (Opti-Fix No 0) broke 11 years after primary replacement. Revision of both components followed

Fig. 11.43 On the right hip exchange of the polyethylene was required because of wear, 13 years after insertion. Left hip after revision

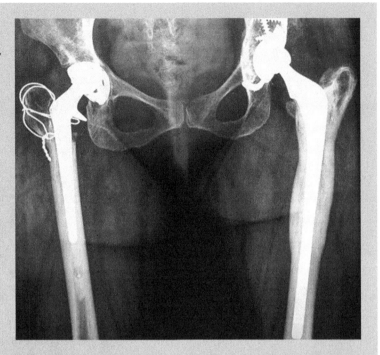

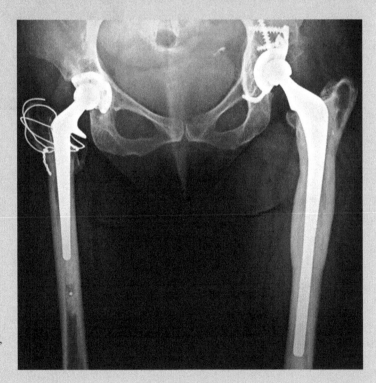

Fig. 11.44 Final radiograph, 19 years after primary replacements

References

1. Roidis NT, Pollalis A, Hartofilakidis G (2013) Total hip arthroplasty in young females with congenital dislocation of the hip, radically improves their long-term quality of life. J Arthroplasty 28(7):1206–1211

2. Engesaeter IO, Lehmann T, Laborie LB, Lie SA, Rosendahl K, Engesaeter LB (2011) Total hip replacement in young adults with hip dysplasia: age at diagnosis, previous treatment, quality of life, and validation of diagnoses reported to the Norwegian Arthroplasty Register between 1987 and 2007. Acta Orthop 82(2):149–154

3. Hartofilakidis G, Babis GC (2009) Congenital disease of the hip. Clin Orthop Relat Res 467(2):578–579; discussion 580–581

4. Hartofilakidis G, Karachalios T (2004) Total hip arthroplasty for congenital hip disease. J Bone Joint Surg Am 86-A(2):242–250

5. Hartofilakidis G, Karachalios T, Karachalios G (2005) The 20-year outcome of the Charnley arthroplasty in younger and older patients. Clin Orthop Relat Res 434:177–182

6. Hartofilakidis G, Karachalios T, Stamos KG (2000) Epidemiology, demographics, and natural history of congenital hip disease in adults. Orthopedics 23(8): 823–827

7. Hartofilakidis G, Yiannakopoulos CK, Babis GC (2008) The morphologic variations of low and high hip dislocation. Clin Orthop Relat Res 466(4): 820–824

8. Karachalios T, Hartofilakidis G (2010) Congenital hip disease in adults: terminology, classification, preoperative planning and management. J Bone Joint Surg Br 92(7):914–921

Conclusive Messages

- Two types of hip osteoarthritis (OA) are recognised: idiopathic, in which the underlying cause is unknown, and secondary, when the predisposing cause is well known.
- Idiopathic OA is classified into two types: eccentric, which is characterised by a rapid deterioration, and concentric, which has a better prognosis because of its slow deterioration.
- Femoroacetabular impingement (FAI) has also been referred to as a cause of early OA of the hip. However, clinical confirmation to support the hypothesis that FAI cause early OA is still lacking.
- The most suitable term for the entire spectrum of deformities of the hip, already present at birth, is "congenital hip disease".
- We have recognised three main types of CHD of increasing severity: A, dysplasia; B, low dislocation; C, high dislocation.
- Low dislocation is subdivided in B1 subtype (extended coverage of the true acetabulum by the false acetabulum) and B2 subtype (limited coverage). High dislocation is subdivided in subtypes C1 and C2, depending on the presence or the absence of a false acetabulum.
- Congenital hip disease is the most common cause of secondary OA of the hip in young adults.
- Approximately 90 % of patients with CHD are women.
- Dysplasia, low dislocation and high dislocation in adults appear as the evolutions of dysplasia, subluxation and complete dislocation in infancy.
- The term "subluxation" in adults is inappropriate because it simply refers to the degree of displacement of the femoral head, without defining the underlying pathology.
- Conservative measures in early stages of OA due to CHD include the administration of simple analgesics in conjunction with weight reduction and physiotherapy.
- Osteotomies, after the introduction of THR, have limited indications.
- Currently, total hip replacement (THR) is the treatment of choice for patients with CHD.
- Main indications for THR are:
  - The intensity of pain
  - The degree of disability
  - Psychological consequences
- The simply the fact that new prostheses and methods were developed and surgical experience has increased is not a valid reason to rush for surgery.
- Usually patients with CHD need THR at the third decade of their life.
- There are cases that surgery can be postponed for a few or more years. However, any consequences of a postponed surgery should be considered.
- Patients' age is seriously considered. The likelihood of revision surgery in young patients is most possible. However, age only cannot be a prohibitive factor for depriving these patients of enjoyment in the course of the best and more productive years of their lives.

G. Hartofilakidis et al., *Congenital Hip Disease in Adults*,
DOI 10.1007/978-88-470-5492-9_12, © Springer-Verlag Italia 2014

- Preoperative assessment with the use of 3D-CT scans is recommended in borderline cases, for the distinction between dysplastic hips and hips with low dislocation of B1 subtype and between hips with low dislocation of B2 subtype and hips with high dislocation of C1 subtype.
- THR, especially in patients with low and high dislocations, is a demanding operation. The use of special techniques and implants is mandatory.
- The transtrochanteric approach (TTA) is essential in cases with low and high dislocation, and all orthopaedic surgeons should know this approach.
- The benefits from TTA far overweight the complications arising from it.
- Restoration of the normal centre of rotation is essential for the joint biomechanics and survival of the prosthesis.
- When cementless components are used, at least 70–80 % coverage of the implant with bone is needed. If this cannot be obtained, the cotyloplasty technique is recommended or a modified technique using cementless components.
- When cemented technique is used for the reconstruction of the acetabulum, full coverage of implant by host bone is needed.
- For the reconstruction of a straight femur with narrow canal, cemented special CDH stems can provide better fixation.

- Shortening of the leg at the level of the neck of the femur is simple and uneventful.
- We do not favour shortening at the femoral diaphysis. An intraoperative creation of an artificial fracture may cause undesirable complications.
- Proper postoperative management, adjusted to the particularities of the surgical technique, is important.
- While reporting THR outcomes in patients with CHD, mixing results of the three types may lead to statistical bias.
- Short term results are unreliable.
- Follow-up for lifetime of patients with THR and revision on time is of fundamental importance.
- Since osteolysis and wear are initially symptomless, revision is a matter for the surgeon to decide.
- Though revision operation is undesirable for the patient and raises the financial cost, it can be successful if it is performed early before extensive bone destruction occurs.
- Quality of life of young female patients with congenitally dislocated hips radically improves after THR.
- Even patients who underwent several revisions had the opportunity to enjoy life for a reasonable period of time with functional improvement and without pain.

Index

A

Abduction devices, 30
Abductor force, 67
Abductor lever arm, 63, 67
Abductor mechanism, 63
Acetabular angle, 33
Acetabular component, 56, 64, 65, 67, 69, 70, 77, 78, 80–84, 90, 92, 113, 114, 116, 117, 119, 124, 134, 138, 141, 142, 144, 145, 149
Acetabular floor, 1, 67, 70, 126
Acetabular fossa, 1, 2, 16
Acetabular notch, 1, 65, 68
Acetabuloplasty technique, 67
Age, 3, 29, 47, 53, 83, 87, 114, 131, 165
Anatomical abnormalities, 3, 12, 15–17, 39, 79, 80, 84
Ankylosis, 78, 79
Anteversion, 16, 22, 56, 65, 67, 70, 73, 78
Arthroscopy, 5, 7
Artificial joint, 53, 113
Aseptic loosening, 82–84

B

Bilateral, 11, 29, 32, 38–42, 47, 55, 87, 90, 95, 104, 107, 110, 138, 143, 145, 148, 151, 153, 159
Biomechanical patterns, 33
Biomechanics, 63, 166
Body deformations, 131
Bone cuts, 57, 59
Bone deficiencies, 20
Bone loss, 123–125, 128
Bone stock, 22, 54, 56, 65, 68, 82, 113, 123–125, 128
Bony coverage, 67, 84, 109
Borderline cases, 19, 20, 22–24, 58, 60, 166
Brooker, A.F., 78
B1 subtype, 22, 25, 27, 60, 165, 166
B2 subtype, 22, 25, 27, 60, 79, 165, 166
Bulk structural autogenous graft, 68, 72
Busch-Schneider cages, 124

C

Capital drop, 17
Cartilaginous anlage, 1
Causes of failure, 117

CDH prosthesis, 84
Cement(ed), 64, 67–70, 73, 81, 83, 94, 102, 103, 107, 114, 116, 123–125, 127, 133, 136, 143, 166
Cement-in-cement, 124
Cementless cup, 65, 84
Cement mantle, 70, 73, 81
Central-edge angle of Wiberg, 33
Charnley deepening reamer, 67
Charnley low-friction arthroplasty (LFA), 78, 123, 131
Charnley offset-bore socket, 83
CHD in infants, 30
Chiari osteotomy, 42
Circumferential segmental defects, 82
Classification, 7, 11–27, 125, 128
Comminuted fracture, 67, 70
Complete dislocation, 30, 41, 80, 165
Complications, 12, 45, 46, 53, 54, 57, 63, 64, 73, 77–84, 124, 158, 166
Concentric, 3, 5, 6, 165
Congenital dislocation of the hip, 12, 14, 74, 84, 90, 94, 95, 102, 107, 166
Congenital displacement, 12
Conservative management, 45–51
Cortical perforation, 77
Cotyloplasty, 67–72, 81–83, 90, 92, 94, 95, 104, 107, 126, 131, 136, 138, 143, 145, 148, 149, 166
Cross-linked polyethylene, 83
Crowe classification, 15, 17, 19, 20, 22
C1 subtype, 22, 26, 27, 83, 165, 166
C2 subtype, 22, 26, 27, 83, 165

D

D'Antonio classification, 128
3D-CT scan, 1, 20, 22–26, 41, 42, 58, 60, 166
Defective union, 78
Definitely loose, 116, 123
Deformed femoral diaphysis, 77
Demographics, 29–43
Developmental displacement, 14
Developmental dysplasia of the hip, 14, 80
Disability, 11, 38, 45, 56, 131, 156

Dislocation(s), 5, 12, 29, 51, 53, 63, 77, 87, 114, 131, 165
Distal shortening of the femoral diaphysis, 73
Drop foot, 78
Dysplasia, 14–17, 19, 20, 22, 23, 27, 29–31, 34, 56, 60, 80, 92, 138, 148, 165

E
Early symptoms, 30
Eccentric OA, 3, 4, 7, 165
Eftekhar classification, 15, 17, 19
Epidemiology, 29–43
Estok and Harris classification, 125, 128
Expansile osteolysis, 83
External rotators, 70

F
Failure mechanisms, 116
Failure rate, 69, 78, 80, 83
False acetabulum, 15, 16, 18, 19, 22, 25–27, 33, 38, 40, 54, 60, 64, 65, 68, 83, 165
Femoral canal, 58, 72, 73, 77, 124
Femoral component, 57, 63, 65, 70, 81, 84, 114, 123–125, 138, 158
Femoral fracture, 77, 78, 124
Femoral nerves, 73, 77, 78
Femoral shortening, 22, 58, 61, 70, 72, 73, 87, 92, 166
Femoroacetabular impingement (FAI), 5, 7, 11, 165
Fibrous union, 78, 136, 139
Flexion deformity, 53, 77
Follow-up of patients with total hip replacement (THR), 113
Functional improvement, 131, 166

G
Girdlestone, 83
Gold standard, 54
Greater trochanter, 58, 63, 65, 73, 87, 124, 126, 128

H
Harris-Galante cup, 102
Harris technique, 72
Hartofilakidis classification, 15–17, 19, 20, 22, 27
Head-neck junction, 15, 19, 58
Height of the dislocation, 17, 58, 61, 94, 95, 102, 107, 143, 151
Heterotopic ossification, 78, 79
High dislocation, 16, 17, 19–22, 24, 26, 27, 30, 38–40, 53, 55, 57, 59, 60, 63, 65–69, 71, 77–84, 87, 92, 94, 95, 100, 102, 107, 109, 114, 122, 131, 143, 145, 151, 154, 158, 165, 166
High hip centre, 77
Hip loads, 64
Hip pain, 11
Hohmann retractors, 65, 68

Hybrid, 68, 78, 92, 101, 102, 104, 107, 110, 122, 151, 152, 154–159
Hypoplastic femoral diaphysis, 77, 81

I
Idiopathic OA, 3–7, 29, 100, 109, 165
Incidence of CHD, 29
Inclination, 31, 32, 53, 65, 67, 78, 84
Indication, 7, 11, 12, 14, 45, 46, 53–61, 165
Indications for THR, 12
Infant hips, 15
Infection, 77, 78, 158, 160
Intermediate dislocation, 17, 19
Internal fixation, 78
Interobserver reliability, 20
Intra-articular corticosteroids, 45
Intraobserver reliability, 20

J
Joint capsule, 65, 68

K
Kerboull classification, 15, 17, 19

L
Labrum, 1, 5, 7
Leg-length, 64, 94, 107, 131, 143, 145, 151, 154, 156, 158
Leg-length discrepancy, 38, 94, 107, 131
Leg-lengthening, 22, 77
Lesser trochanter, 16, 61, 63, 70, 72
Lever arm of the abductors, 67
Lever arm of the body weight, 64, 67
Lexer chisel, 67
Ligamentum teres, 1
Limp(ing), 3, 4, 11, 13, 32, 33, 37, 38, 53–55, 131, 132, 136–138, 143, 145, 148, 151, 154, 156, 158
Linear osteolysis, 83, 123
Liner(s), 79, 83, 110, 117, 122, 151, 153
Locking mechanism, 83, 113
Long-term, 5, 69, 78–80, 82, 83, 123, 131
Loosening, 64, 65, 78, 82–84, 95, 96, 108, 113, 116, 117, 121, 123–125, 131, 133, 136, 138, 142
Lordosis, 38
Low-back pain, 38
Low dislocation, 16–20, 22–25, 27, 30, 35, 37, 42, 51, 56, 57, 60, 65, 68, 69, 77–81, 87, 89, 104, 107, 110, 114, 121, 125, 126, 131, 136, 138, 145, 148, 154, 156, 158, 165, 166

M
Marginal osteophytes, 16, 33
McMurray, 14, 46, 50, 51, 104
Medialisation, 68

Medialisation of the cup, 77
Megaprosthesis, 97, 113
Metal shell, 83, 117
Mid-term radiographic results, 83
Migration, 3, 16, 17, 30, 116, 123
Modern cementing techniques, 73
Modular metal-backed cementless prosthesis, 117
Morselised graft, 70

N
Narrow canal, 69, 166
Narrow diaphysis, 16
Natural history, 7, 29–43
Neck-shaft angle, 33
Neonatal hip dislocation, 29
Neonatal hip dysplasia, 29
Neonatal hip instability, 29
Nerve damage, 77, 78
Nerve palsy, 77, 78, 98
Neurological complications, 77
Non-steroidal anti-inflammatory drugs
    (NSAIDs), 45
Normal hip, 1–3, 20, 31, 33
Norwegian Arthroplasty Registry, 77

O
OA of the hip, 3–9, 11, 12, 14, 29, 34, 165
Obturator artery, 1
Offset-bore cup, 67, 71, 83, 90, 94, 95, 107
Offset of the hip joint, 2
Opti-Fix cup, 107
Opti-Fix stem, 107
Osseous containment, 65
Osteochondroplasty, 5, 7
Osteolysis, 65, 83, 84, 113, 116, 117, 121,
    123, 134, 144, 166

P
Paproski classification, 125
Pathogenesis, 14
Pelvic inclination, 53
Pelvic osteotomies, 11, 45, 46
Penetration, 70, 124, 133
Periacetabular osteolysis, 84
Periosteum, 67, 70
Periprosthetic osteolysis, 65
Physiotherapy, 45, 53, 165
Porous metal augments, 124
Positioning, 65, 67
Postoperative care, 78
Preoperative assessment, 7, 53–61, 166
Preoperative diagnosis, 77, 78
Probably loose, 116, 119, 123
Protrusio acetabuli, 63
Protrusion, 68, 124, 126, 128
Proximal shortening, 61, 87

Psoas tendon, 70
Psychological status, 53, 55

R
Radiographic indices, 33
Radiolucent line, 116, 123
Reattachment of the trochanter, 63, 66, 78
Reconstruction of the acetabulum, 65–67, 69, 71,
    81–83, 94, 166
Reconstruction of the femur, 69–74, 84, 94
Restoration of the normal centre of rotation, 63, 64, 67,
    166
Result(s), 7, 11, 12, 15, 17, 22, 45, 46, 56, 65, 66, 69, 73,
    77–84, 87, 88, 113, 123, 132, 138, 158, 166
Resultant force, 67
Revision, 12, 63, 74, 77–81, 83, 90, 91, 95–99, 105, 106,
    108, 110, 113–128, 131, 133, 134, 136–138, 141,
    142, 145, 158, 161, 162, 165, 166
Revision rate, 78, 81

S
Schanz, 14, 21, 46, 51, 58, 92, 94, 100
Sciatic nerves, 73
Scoliosis, 38
Secondary OA, 3, 5, 7, 11–14, 29, 32, 34, 42, 45, 51, 87,
    123, 165
Segmental defects, 56, 82
Shearing forces, 64
Shenton's line, 30
Short-term results, 78
Simple analgesics, 45, 165
Stamos technique, 67, 72
Statistical bias, 22, 83, 166
Structural grafts, 68, 69, 72
Subluxation, 15–17, 22, 27, 30, 33, 35, 42, 80, 165
Subsidence, 123
Subtrochanteric shortening of the femoral
    diaphysis, 73
Survival rate, 22, 78, 82, 84
Symptomatic slow-acting drugs in OA
    (SYSADOA), 45, 51

T
Teardrop, 2, 15, 25, 58, 65, 84
Technical difficulties, 14, 63, 123
Templates, 58
Terminology, 7, 11–17
Timely revision, 113
Transtrochanteric approach (TTA), 63, 64, 166
Transverse ligament, 1
Trendelenburg gait, 66, 78
Trochanteric non-union, 63, 77
Trochanteric osteotomy, 13, 14, 35, 45, 47–49, 57,
    63, 64, 78, 87, 102, 110, 119, 128
True acetabulum, 15, 16, 18, 19, 22, 25–27, 60, 64,
    65, 68, 69, 81, 165

U
Unilateral, 5, 7, 64, 68

V
Valgus osteotomy, 45, 46
Varus intertrochanteric osteotomy, 45, 47, 48, 57

W
Wagner type designs, 73, 128
Wear of polyethylene, 65, 79, 103, 113, 116,
    121, 134, 153

Wear of the polyethylene acetabular liner, 79
Weight bearing surface, 33
Wide exposure, 63–65, 87

Y
Young patients, 7, 53, 113, 124, 165

Z
Zones I and II of DeLee and Charnley, 83

Printed in the United States
By Bookmasters